THIRD EDITION

STATISTICS FOR NURSING

A Practical Approach

ELIZABETH HEAVEY, PhD, RN, CNM

Professor of Nursing
SUNY College at Brockport
Brockport, New York

JONES & BARTLETT
LEARNING

World Headquarters
Jones & Bartlett Learning
5 Wall Street
Burlington, MA 01803
978-443-5000
info@jblearning.com
www.jblearning.com

Jones & Bartlett Learning books and products are available through most bookstores and online booksellers. To contact Jones & Bartlett Learning directly, call 800-832-0034, fax 978-443-8000, or visit our website, www.jblearning.com.

14399-7

Production Credits
VP, Product Management: David D. Cella
Director of Product Management: Amanda Martin
Product Manager: Rebecca Stephenson
Product Assistant: Christina Freitas
Senior Vendor Manager: Sara Kelly
Senior Marketing Manager: Jennifer Scherzay
Product Fulfillment Manager: Wendy Kilborn

Composition and Project Management: S4Carlisle Publishing Services
Cover Design: Kristin E. Parker
Rights & Media Specialist: Wes DeShano
Media Development Editor: Troy Liston
Cover Image (Title Page, Part Opener, Chapter Opener):
  © sinemaslow/iStock/Getty Images Plus/Getty
Printing and Binding: LSC Communications, Harrisonburg
Cover Printing: LSC Communications, Harrisonburg

Library of Congress Cataloging-in-Publication Data
Names: Heavey, Elizabeth, author.
Title: Statistics for nursing : a practical approach / Elizabeth Heavey,
    Ph.D., R.N., C.N.M., Professor of Nursing, SUNY College at Brockport.
Description: Third edition. | Burlington, MA : Jones & Bartlett Learning,
    [2019] | Includes index.
Identifiers: LCCN 2017054187 | ISBN 9781284142013 (paperback)
Subjects: LCSH: Nursing--Statistical methods.
Classification: LCC RT68 .H43 2019 | DDC 610.73072/7--dc23 LC record available at https://lccn.loc.gov/2017054187

6048

Printed in the United States of America
22 21 20 19 18   10 9 8 7 6 5 4 3

DEDICATION

This book is dedicated to my RN to BSN students, who remind me every day how much effort, persistence, and determination it takes to return to school while balancing work, family, and professional responsibilities. Your feedback and willingness to challenge yourselves, despite the many obligations and responsibilities you have in your lives, inspires me. I have watched so many of you arrive in class tired, very unsure, anxious, and stressed about taking statistics, and yet you persevere. You put your best foot forward, tentatively realizing that, though it isn't easy, you have the capacity to master this content and reach your goals. Sometimes you stumble, but you get back up and try again and because of that, I have watched you accomplish so much in all avenues of your lives. It makes me so proud to watch you figure out difficult content, develop understanding of how this really will have an impact on your patient care, and grow as nurses and individuals. Nothing makes me happier than to be part of your success, to watch you walk across the stage at graduation, ready for the next challenge in your educational and professional path. I watch your families, so proud of all that you are and all that you do. I watch your children realize they too can dream big and succeed because they have watched you do just that. It is a joy and privilege to work with each of you, and just like you, I keep trying to grow and improve. So here is my third try at this book, and I hope you find that listening to my students has helped make this edition even better—because you are the reason it exists in the first place.

Beth

CONTENTS

INTRODUCTION   IX
ACKNOWLEDGMENTS   XI

CHAPTER 1: INTRODUCTION TO STATISTICS AND
LEVELS OF MEASUREMENT   1

Introduction   2
Population Versus Sample   4
Quantitative Versus Qualitative   4
Independent Versus Dependent Variables   5
Continuous Versus Categorical Variables   6
Levels of Measurement   6
Summary   11
Review Questions   12

CHAPTER 2: PRESENTING DATA   19

Frequency Distributions   21
Percentages   22
Bar Charts   23
Histograms   28
Line Graphs   29
Scatterplots   29
Box and Whiskers Plot   30
Summary   31
Review Questions   31

CHAPTER 3: DESCRIPTIVE STATISTICS, PROBABILITY,
AND MEASURES OF CENTRAL TENDENCY   41

Descriptive Statistics: Properties of Variables   43
Measures of Central Tendency   43
Range and Sample Standard Deviation   44
Calculating the Standard Deviation   45
Using a Box and Whiskers Plot to Display Central Tendency and Range   47

Moving Forward: Inferential Statistics   51

Frequency Distributions Versus Probability Distributions   51

The Normal Distribution   54

Skewed Distributions   56

Summary   57

Review Questions   58

CHAPTER 4: MEASURING DATA   63

Feasibility   65

Validity   65

Reliability   66

Screening Tests   68

Sensitivity   69

Specificity   69

Positive Predictive Value of a Screen   71

Negative Predictive Value   73

Efficiency   74

Summary   74

Review Questions   75

CHAPTER 5: SAMPLING METHODS   83

Sampling Methods   84

Probability Sampling   85

Sampling Error Versus Sampling Bias   86

Sampling Distributions   87

Nonprobability Sampling   90

Inclusion and Exclusion Criteria   92

Sample Size   92

Summary   93

Review Questions   93

CHAPTER 6: GENERATING THE RESEARCH IDEA   99

Hypothesis Testing   100

Statistical Significance   102

Statistical Significance Versus Clinical Significance   104

How Does the Test Statistic Compare to the Null Hypothesis?   106

Applying the Decision Rule   107

Test Statistics and Corresponding p-Values   107

Summary   107

Review Questions   108

Chapter 7: Sample Size, Effect Size, and Power   113

Effect Size   114
Type Two Error   117
A Quick Review of Type One and Type Two Errors   118
Sample Size   119
Summary   121
Review Questions   121

Chapter 8: Chi-Square   127

Chi-Square (X^2) Test   128
The Null and Alternative Hypotheses   128
2×2 Table   128
Degrees of Freedom   129
Statistical Significance   129
Direction of the Relationship   129
When Not to Use Chi-Square: Assumptions and Special Cases   132
Summary   135
Review Questions   136

Chapter 9: Student t-Test   145

The Student t-Test   146
The Null and Alternative Hypotheses   152
Statistical Significance   152
Degrees of Freedom for Student t-Tests   152
Summary   160
Review Questions   161

Chapter 10: Analysis of Variance (ANOVA)   171

Comparing More Than Two Samples   172
The Null and Alternative Hypotheses   172
Degrees of Freedom   174
Statistical Significance   174
Appropriate Use of ANOVA   175
Repeat-Measures ANOVA   176
Summary   181
Review Questions   181

Chapter 11: Correlation Coefficients   191

Looking for a Relationship in One Sample   192
The Null and Alternative Hypotheses   192

Selecting the Best Correlation Test to Use   193
Direction of the Relationship   193
Sample Size   194
Strength of the Relationship   194
Statistical Significance   194
Appropriate Use of Correlation Coefficients   195
More Uses for Pearson's *r*   195
Summary   198
Review Questions   200

CHAPTER 12: REGRESSION ANALYSIS   207

Quantifying an Association   208
Summary   239
Review Questions   239

CHAPTER 13: RELATIVE RISK, ODDS RATIO, AND ATTRIBUTABLE RISK   249

Epidemiology   251
Study Designs Used in Epidemiology   251
Attributable Risk   265
Summary   266
Review Questions   267

APPENDIX A: TABLES FOR REFERENCE   277
APPENDIX B: WORKING WITH SMALL SAMPLES   287
REFERENCES   291
EPILOGUE   295
INDEX   297

INTRODUCTION

When the first edition of *Statistics for Nursing: A Practical Approach* came out, I was very happy to hear from many nurses about how useful it was in making statistics accessible for anyone just beginning to work with these concepts. They also had some very helpful suggestions, much like my own students, who provided the motivation and feedback that helped create the first edition of the book. I also heard from quite a few of you in DNP programs that the book was helpful to get you started as well. Wonderful! I am thrilled to be a part of nurses going on into advanced practice!

In this third edition, I have again acted on the feedback from students, and I have included even more practice questions at the end of each chapter, giving you more opportunities to practice, practice, practice. A whole new test bank provides instructors the opportunity to use the older questions as practice quizzes, which also provides students with additional feedback and practice. I have also provided new research article reviews with practice questions within the analysis chapters of the text. Teaching from the text myself has given me the opportunity to identify areas where students needed additional support, so I have added content like decision trees and tables showing the different tests and how to differentiate which one is appropriate. However, I have stayed true to the original premise of the text, which is that all of this is at an introductory level, without a lot of ancillary information to confuse you.

If you are teaching from this text at an undergraduate level, it is perfectly appropriate to skip the regression chapter; the rest of the content from the book will still work fine. You can also include it if it is appropriate for your students or course. As with the previous edition, the

"From the Statistician" features examine some of the chapter concepts in greater detail. A new "From the Statistician" feature in Chapter 13 provides additional background about confidence intervals. These features are set apart from the rest of the text and are available for students who prefer a more mathematical approach or want to have a better understanding of "why." Students who want to stick with the clinically applied information can skip these sections without experiencing problems in understanding the essential content.

The third edition of *Statistics for Nursing* also includes updated recorded lectures with closed captioning available and computer application updates. I have started using skeletal notes when I teach this class, and I provide these for my students to use in each chapter; these notes are included for all students as well. They provide an outline for note taking and helpful graphics to fill in, thus promoting student engagement with the content rather than just their passive printing of PowerPoint slides.

I would love to hear from any of you who use the new content and supports in the third edition of this text. What are your thoughts? Did these new resources help you? Do you have any other ideas for useful learning tools? Send me a quick email and help me make this material even better.

I hope you find the third edition of *Statistics for Nursing* helpful and that you continue on your quest to becoming a nurse who understands statistics! You never know where it may take you someday. I certainly didn't!

All the best,
Beth

Acknowledgments

This book is the product of the combined effort of many individuals who were gracious enough to contribute their time, knowledge, and effort.

Brendan Heavey is the contributing author for all of the "From the Statistician" features in the text and has developed the computer application content for Excel. Brendan has a statistical knowledge significantly beyond my own and spent many hours writing, rewriting, and explaining concepts to make sure my simplified explanations were technically correct. I am ever grateful not only for his statistical contributions to the text but also for his interest in and support of the project from the early proposal days. He is an incredibly gifted human being. I am proud to call him my brother.

Dr. Renee Biedlingmaier, a former star student and now valued colleague, shares her experience working with small samples in the new Appendix B for this book. Several of the DNP instructors asked for a brief overview of this challenging topic. Her expertise and willingness to share it with our students enhance the book, and her contribution is greatly appreciated.

The RN to BSN faculty members at SUNY Brockport believe this content is essential to the knowledge and future success of nurses, and they have supported the inclusion of the course for all RN to BSN students in our program. Thank you! My colleagues, Dr. Biedlingmaier and Professor Bingham, have been graciously willing to teach the class with me and have helped solidify student support content and data collection for evaluation of new material.

Ms. Shelby Brown, one of our traditional nursing students, dedicated many hours to helping me input content and complete computer work efficiently. Her effort and skill are greatly appreciated!

Many other undergraduate and graduate students emailed me from afar with feedback and thoughts about the book. I always enjoy hearing how this book has had an impact on your understanding and your career, as well as your suggestions for improvement. Thank you for taking the time to share these ideas with me.

Thank you also to all the instructors who are using the book and letting me know how well it is working in your classrooms. You inspire and encourage me with all of your great ideas and dedication to student learning.

Thank you to the publishing team at Jones & Bartlett Learning, who saw the potential in the first edition before I did and helped make it happen, and then came back for more!

As always, my heartfelt gratitude goes to my family and friends, who loved and supported me throughout this project. I would not be where I am today without all of you. Thank you for all the hours spent watching swim meets, hosting sleepovers, and climbing rock walls and kayaking on camping trips; the homecooked meals, quiet hugs, and heartfelt phone calls; and the belief in me no matter what crazy plan I come up with next. I will always be grateful for each of you.

And to my children, Gabrielle and Nathaniel, you are the reason behind it all, why every day matters and making the most of it counts. Watching you grow into the young people that you are has been a journey that has involved very little sleep but has brought me tremendous joy. You have made me more humble, reflective, forgiving, and determined to have an impact on the world you will inherit from our generation. Being your mother puts the meaning in everything that I do. I love you to the moon and the stars, to infinity and beyond and back again, forever and ever.

Thank you all,
Beth

INTRODUCTION TO STATISTICS AND LEVELS OF MEASUREMENT

HOW TO FIGURE THINGS OUT.

OBJECTIVES

By the end of this chapter students will be able to:

- State the question that statistics is always trying to answer.

- Define the empirical method.

- Compare quantitative and qualitative variables.

- Differentiate a population from a sample and a statistic from a parameter, giving an example of each.

- Explain the difference between an independent and a dependent variable, citing examples of each.

- Identify continuous and categorical variables accurately.

- Distinguish the four levels of measurement, and describe each.

- Apply several beginning-level statistical techniques to further develop understanding of the concepts discussed in this chapter.

KEY TERMS

Categorical variable
A variable that has a finite number of classification groups or categories, which are usually qualitative in nature.

Continuous variable
A variable that has an infinite number of potential values, with the value being measured falling somewhere on a continuum containing in-between values.

Dependent variable
The outcome variable or final result.

Empirical method
A way of gathering information through systematic observation and experimentation.

Estimate
A preliminary approximation.

Independent variable
A variable measured or controlled by the experimenter; the variable that is thought to affect the outcome.

Interval data
Data whose categories are exhaustive, exclusive, and rank-ordered, with equally spaced intervals.

Nominal data
Data that indicates a difference only, with categories that are exhaustive and exclusive but not rank-ordered.

Ordinal data
Data whose categories are exhaustive, exclusive, and rank-ordered.

Parameter
Descriptive result for the whole group.

Population
The whole group.

Probability
The likelihood that an outcome will occur.

Qualitative measure
A measure that describes or characterizes an attribute.

Quantitative measure
A measure that reflects a numeric amount.

Ratio data
Data whose categories are exhaustive, exclusive, and rank-ordered with equally spaced intervals and a point at which the variable does not exist.

Sample
A group selected from the population.

Statistic
An estimate derived from a sample.

Variable
The changing characteristic being measured.

INTRODUCTION

So here you are. You've worked hard, you are in nursing school, and you are ready to begin. But wait! Why do you have to take statistics? Why do you need to understand all those numbers and equations when you are a nurse and want to help people?

Most nursing students experience a mild sense of panic when they discover they have to take statistics—or any other kind of math, for that matter. That reaction is common. Here is a calming thought to remember: You already practice statistics, but you just may not know it.

Statistics boils down to doing two things:

- Looking at data
- Applying tests to find out either (1) that what you observe is what you expected or (2) that your observation differs enough from what you expected that you need to change your expectations

You might be convinced that you don't use statistics in your life, so let me give you an example. New York State, where I live, has four seasons. The summer is usually June, July, and August. Fall is September, October, and November. Winter is December, January, and February. And that leaves March, April, and May for the spring. If you walk outside in July and find it to be 80° and humid, you would draw an unspoken conclusion that what you just observed is what you were expecting, and you would put on your sunglasses. However, what if you walk outside in January and find it to be 80° and humid? You would probably be startled, take off your overcoat and boots, and read about global warming. The difference between the weather you expect in winter and what you actually encounter is so different that you might need to change your expectations. You are already practicing statistics without knowing it!

Of course, that day in January might just be a fluke occurrence (a random event), and the temperature could be below freezing again the next day. That is why we need to use the **empirical method**, otherwise known as systematic observation and experimentation. The empirical method allows you to determine whether the temperature observed is *consistently* different from what you expect. To use the empirical method, you need to check the daily temperature on more than one day. So you might decide to monitor the daily temperature for a whole month of winter to see whether readings are consistently different from what you expect in the winter months. In this scenario, you would be using the empirical method to practice statistics (see **Figure 1-1**).

FIGURE 1-1   **Long-Range Winter Forecast for 2017.**

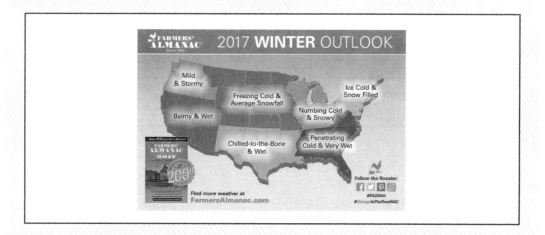

POPULATION VERSUS SAMPLE

To answer questions in research, we need to set up a study of the concepts we're interested in and define multiple **variables**, that is, the changing characteristics being measured. In our example, the temperature is a variable, a measured characteristic. Each variable has an associated **probability** for each of its possible outcomes, that is, how likely it is the outcome will occur. For example, how likely is it that the temperature will be below freezing as opposed to being in the eighties in winter? In your study, you recorded the daily temperature for a winter month, and those readings make up a **sample** of all the daily temperatures in the months of winter. The manner in which you collect your sample is dependent on the purpose of your study (**Figure 1-2**).

A sample is always a subset of a **population**, or an overall group (sometimes referred to as the reference population). In this case, our population includes all the daily temperatures in the winter months, and the subset, or sample, is all the daily temperatures recorded during your month of data collection. If you calculate the average temperature based on this sample

data, you create what is called a **statistic**, which is an **estimate** generated from a sample.

A measured characteristic of a population is called a **parameter**. In our example, if you measured the daily temperature for December, January, and February and then calculated the average temperature, you would be determining a parameter. A really good way to remember the relationships among these four terms is with the following analogy: Statistic is to sample as parameter is to population.

QUANTITATIVE VERSUS QUALITATIVE

While you are collecting the weather data, you may realize that the data can be recorded in several ways. You could write down the actual temperature on that day, which would be a **quantitative measurement**, or you could describe the day as "warm" or "cold," which would be a **qualitative measurement**. A numeric amount or measure is associated with quantitative measurement (such as 80°F), and qualitative measures describe or characterize things (such as, "So darn cold I can't feel my toes").

Be careful with this difference: You can easily get confused. Qualitative variables do not contain quantity information, even if numbers are assigned. The assigned numbers have no quantitative information, rank, or distance. For example, a survey question asks, "What color scrubs are you wearing?" and lists choices numbered 1 to 3. Even if you selected choice 2, neon orange, you do not necessarily have any more scrubs than someone who chooses 1, lime green (although both respondents may want to purchase new scrubs). Even though these qualitative variables have numbers assigned to them, the numbers simply help with coding. The variables are still qualitative.

| FIGURE 1-2 | **Population vs. Sample.** |

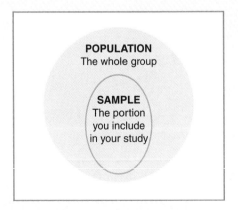

INDEPENDENT VERSUS DEPENDENT VARIABLES

Being as inquisitive as you are, you have probably asked yourself a number of times about a relationship you observe in your patients. For example, you notice that many supportive family members visit Sally Smith after her hip replacement recovery and that she is discharged 3 days after her surgery. Joanne Jones, on the other hand, has no visitors during her hip replacement recovery and is not discharged until day 6. As an observant nurse researcher, you have been wondering how variable x (the **independent variable**, which is measured or controlled by the experimenter) affects variable y (the **dependent variable**, or outcome variable) (**Figure 1-3**). You wonder, does having family support (the independent variable) affect the duration of a hospital stay (the dependent, or outcome, variable)?

To answer this question, you create a study. Obviously, other factors might be involved as well, but in your experiment, you are interested in how family support, the independent variable, affects hospital stay, the dependent variable. If you are correct, then the duration of the hospital stay *depends* on family support. The independent variable can be a suspected causative agent, and the dependent variable is the measured outcome or effect (**Figure 1-4**).

FIGURE 1-3   **Relationship of Independent and Dependent Variables.**

FIGURE 1-4   **Does Family Support Affect the Duration of a Subject's Hospital Stay?**

Note: Additional criteria must be met to say that a variable is causative, so I refer here only to the "suspected" causative agent.

CONTINUOUS VERSUS CATEGORICAL VARIABLES

Some data have an infinite number of potential values, and the value you measure falls somewhere on a continuum containing in-between values. These values are called **continuous variables**. As a nurse, when you measure your patient's temperature, you are measuring a continuous variable. The reading could be 98° or 98.6° or 98.66666°. The infinite possibilities are all quantitative in nature. Actually, the only limit to the measurement is the accuracy of the measuring device. For example, if you have a thermometer that measures only in whole degrees, you will not have as much information as you would using a thermometer that measures to the one-thousandth of a degree.

Continuous variables can be contrasted with **categorical variables**, sometimes called discrete variables, which have a finite number of classification groups, or categories, that are usually qualitative in nature. For example, as part of your research you may need to collect information about your patients' racial background. The choices available are African American, Native American, Caucasian, Asian, Latino, mixed race, and other. Race is an example of a categorical variable, a measurement that is restricted to a specific value and does not have any fractional or in-between values. When you read a study, the demographic information about the sample involved usually contains quite a few categorical variables including marital status, gender, race, geographic region, educational level, language spoken, smoking status, and so on.

Let's look at an example where we can see both types of variables in a study. If you were reading a public health study examining statewide variation in population estimates you might have the information in **Figure 1-5** available. Your sample was collected and reported about five states, so the state becomes one of the demographic variables you will want to report. Note that "state" is a categorical/qualitative variable: It just tells you the location of the sample subject and does not include any quantitative information. You also record the state population, which is a continuous/quantitative variable where the value can fall anywhere within the range of population values.

LEVELS OF MEASUREMENT

Let's say that your interest in the relationship between family support (the independent variable) and duration of stay (the dependent variable) is extensive enough that you apply for a program at your hospital that includes a small research fellowship. You win the fellowship and proceed to collect data about each patient admitted to your orthopedic unit for hip replacement over a 3-month period. The study protocol calls for you to complete the usual admission forms and then for patients to complete a short survey about perceived family support. After your institutional review board approves your

FIGURE 1-5   **Projected Populations by State.**

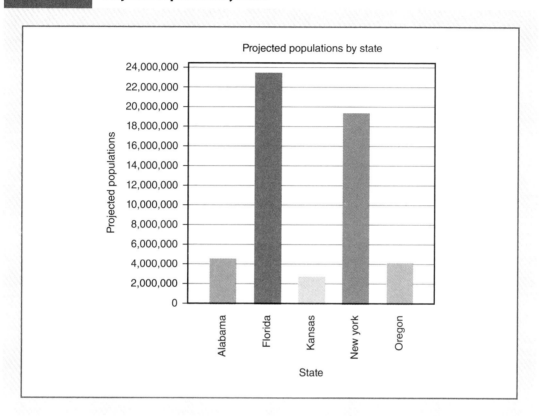

Projected populations by state

Reproduced from CDC. (n.d). Population Projections, United States, 2004–2030, by state, age and sex. CDC WONDER Online Database, September 2005. Accessed at http://wonder
.cdc.gov/population-projections.html on Apr 4, 2017.

study, you begin. The level of measurement of your data determines what type of analysis you are able to perform in your study, so let's look at the different types and what makes each level unique.

Your first survey question asks the patient's gender (male, female, other). The data you gather for this question is an example of **nominal data**; it simply indicates a difference between the three answers. One is neither greater than nor less than the other, and they are not in any particular order. Also, the categories are exclusive and exhaustive; that is, the patient cannot answer "both" or "neither." Asking about

FROM THE STATISTICIAN *Brendan Heavey*

What Is a Statistic?

As a student of statistics, you will run into questions regarding parameters and statistics all the time. Determining the difference between the two can be difficult. To get a concrete idea of the difference, let's look at an example. According to the Bureau of Labor Statistics, registered nurses constitute the largest healthcare occupation, with 2.7 million jobs nationwide. Because this text is primarily designed for nursing students, let's use this number for our example.

Let's say that you are a consultant working for a fledgling company that is planning to make scrubs for nurses. Let's call this company Carol's Nursing Scrubs, Inc. Scrubs at Carol's come in small, medium, and large. The company offers all kinds of styles and prints, but the underlying sizes are intended to remain the same. Carol just received her first bit of seed money to mass-produce 20,000 pairs of scrubs. Carol, an overly demanding boss, wants the medium-size scrubs to fit as many nurses nationwide as possible. To make that happen, she needs to know the average height and weight of nurses nationwide, so she has instructed you to conduct a nationwide poll. She thinks you should ask every nurse in the country his or her height and weight and then calculate the average of all the numbers you get.

Now, you are an intelligent, well-grounded employee who's in demand everywhere and working for Carol only because her health plan comes with a sweet gym membership and you get a company car. You realize it would be pretty difficult to set up a nationwide poll and ask all the nurses in the country for their height and weight. Even if you tried a mass mailing, the data returned to you would be filled with so many incompletes and errors that it wouldn't be trustworthy.

So what are you to do? Your first instinct might be to respond to your boss by saying, "Geez, Carol, that's so absurd and impossible I don't even know where I'd start," and then finish your day on the golf range. After this course, however, you'll be not only a nurse but a nurse with some training in statistics. You'll be able to deal with this situation more effectively.

Jenna the Statistical Nursing Guru (you):	Carol, I recommend we take a few *samples* of nurses nationwide and *survey* them rather than attempting to contact every nurse in the country. Then we could *estimate* the true average height and weight based on our samples.
Carol:	How would that work, Jenna?
Jenna:	Well, I'd go down to the University Hospital and poll 30 RNs on their height and weight. Then I'd go to the next state and do the same. My third and final sample would contain 30 RNs from a hospital in Springfield. I'd calculate the average from my total *sample* (90 RNs), which is a *statistic*, and use that to estimate the overall average in the United States, which is a *parameter* of the total *population*.
	You see, Carol, anytime you calculate an estimate with data from a sample or list the data from the sample itself, you calculate a statistic. If you calculate an estimate from data in an entire population, you're calculating a parameter.

the patient's marital status (married, divorced, separated, living together, and other) is another example of nominal data.

Your next survey question asks the patient to rate his or her family support level as low, medium, or high. This question is an example of **ordinal data**. Ordinal data must be exhaustive and exclusive, just like nominal data, but the answers are also rank-ordered. With rank-ordered data, each observation/ category is higher or lower, or better or worse, than another, but you do not know the level of difference between the observations/categories. In this example, a high level of family support indicates a greater quantity of the variable in question than does a moderate or low level of family support

A routine part of admitting each patient also includes a baseline set of vital signs, which you want to include in your survey data. One of the vital signs you check is each subject's temperature. Temperature is an example of **interval data**, which is exhaustive, exclusive, and rank-ordered, and has numerically equal intervals. In this example, the interval is a degree of Fahrenheit. You may also decide you want to look at your survey data by age group and develop the table shown in **Table 1-1**. In this example, age group is interval data; it is

exhaustive, exclusive, and rank-ordered; and each interval is 4 years, so the intervals are all equal.

After recording each patient's temperature, you go on to examine each patient's blood pressure. Blood pressure is an example of **ratio data**, which is exhaustive, exclusive, and rank-ordered, with equal intervals *and* a point at which the variable is absent. (If the blood pressure reading is "absent" in any of your patients, you need to begin CPR!)

If you look at the diagram in **Figure 1-6**, you will see the relationship between the levels of measurement. Each increase in level includes the factors of the previous level, plus it adds another qualifier. Thus, if a variable is at the ratio level, it meets all the criteria for the nominal, ordinal, and interval levels, plus there is a point where it does not exist.

Ratio data is the highest level of measurement you can collect and gives you the greatest number of options for data analysis, but not all variables can be measured at this level. As a general rule of thumb, always collect the highest-level data you can for all your variables, especially your dependent variable. In your study of how family support (the independent variable) affects the duration of hospital stay (the dependent variable), you could have measured the length of hospital stay as short, medium, or long (ordinal) or in the number of actual days (the interval/ ratio level). Obviously, the actual number of days gives you a higher level of measurement. A dependent variable with a higher level of measurement allows for a more robust data analysis. So collect the highest level you can! (See **Figure 1-7**.)

Note: Ordinal data may be quantitative (age group) or qualitative (mild/moderate/severe).

TABLE 1-1	**Number of Patients Surveyed in Each Age Group**

Age Group	Number of Patients
40–44 years	4
45–49 years	22
50–54 years	48
55–59 years	84

FIGURE 1-6   **Relationship between the Levels of Measurement.**

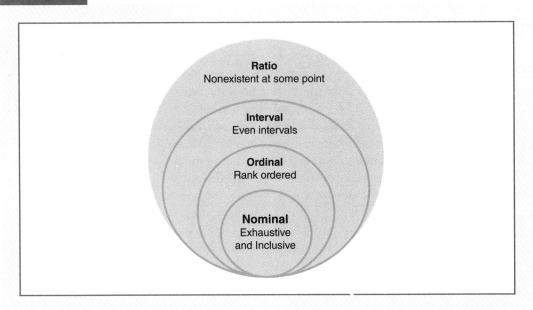

FIGURE 1-7   **The Relationship between Variable Descriptions.**

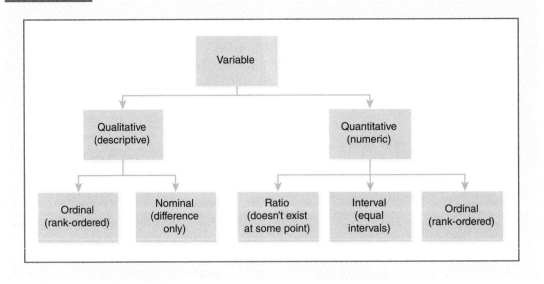

THINK IT THROUGH

How Can I Determine the Level of Measurement of a Variable?

Your study examines placental weight, which is measured in grams. What level of measurement is this variable?

Nominal Level: Ask yourself, does the variable show a difference? Yes, it does, different scores indicate different placental weight. This variable is at least at the nominal level.

If your answer is yes, then go to the next step because the variable may be at a higher level.

Ordinal Level: Is the difference rank-ordered? Yes, a lower score means less placental weight, and a higher score means more placental weight. Your variable is at least at an ordinal level.

If your answer to this question is no, then you do not have the criteria for this level and should identify your variable as the level before, in this case, nominal. If your answer is yes, then go to the next step.

Interval: Does this variable have equal intervals? Yes, each gram is an equal interval. Then your variable is at least interval level.

If your answer to this question is no, then you do not have the criteria for this level and should identify your variable as the level before, in this case, ordinal. If your answer is yes, then go to the next step.

Ratio: Is there a point where the variable can be equal to zero? No, every placenta will have at least some level of mass to it, so the variable will never be equal to zero.

Because your answer to this question is no, you do not have the criteria for this level and should identify your variable as the level before, in this case, interval. If your answer is yes, then you have satisfied the criteria for the highest level of measurement, which is ratio.

Let's look at another example, using the same steps. Your study examines amniotic fluid volume (AFV) measured as minimal, adequate, and excessive. What level measurement is this variable?

Nominal Level: Ask yourself, does the variable show a difference? Yes, it does; different categories indicate different amounts of AFV. This variable is at least at the nominal level.

If your answer is yes, then go to the next step because the variable may be at a higher level.

Ordinal Level: Is the difference rank-ordered? Yes, a person with minimal AFV has less AFV than someone with excessive AFV. Then your variable is at least at the ordinal level.

If your answer to this question is no, then you do not have the criteria for this level and should identify your variable as the level before, in this case, nominal. If your answer is yes, then go to the next step.

Interval: Does this variable have equal intervals? No, we don't know the intervals for these categories, so we can't say they are even.

Because your answer to this question is no, you do not have the criteria for this level and should identify your variable as the level before, in this case, ordinal.

SUMMARY

Talk about exhausting, but you survived! So let's wrap it up here. Statistics really boils down to asking:

- Is what you observe what you expect?
- Or, using the empirical method, have you determined that what you observe is different enough from what you would expect that you need to change your expectations?

Using qualitative (descriptive) and quantitative (numeric) variables, you can assess the impact of independent variables on dependent (outcome) variables. Always collect the highest level of measurement possible, especially for your dependent variable. Doing so gives you the widest range of analysis options when you are ready to "crunch the numbers."

If you understand these concepts, you are ready to move on to the review exercises. If you are still struggling, don't despair. These concepts sometimes take a while to absorb. Read the review questions and then the chapter again, and slowly start to look at the review questions. You will get the hang of statistics; sometimes you just need practice. My students frequently look at me as though I am an alien when I tell them that by the end of the course this chapter will seem really simple. You may not believe it either. As you develop your understanding and apply these concepts, however, they will become clearer, and you too will look back in amazement. You are a statistical genius in the making!

CHAPTER 1 REVIEW QUESTIONS

1. A researcher asks hospitalized individuals about their comfort in a new type of hospital gown. This is an example of what type of data?
   a. ratio
   b. independent
   c. quantitative
   d. qualitative

2. If a researcher is examining how exposure to cigarette ads affects smoking behavior, the cigarette ads are what type of variable?
   a. qualitative
   b. quantitative
   c. dependent
   d. independent

3. A nurse practitioner measures how many times per minute a heart beats when an individual is at rest versus when running. She is measuring the heartbeat at what level of measurement?
   a. interval/ratio
   b. nominal
   c. independent
   d. ordinal

4. If a researcher is examining how exposure to cigarette ads affects smoking behavior, smoking behavior is what type of variable?
   a. ratio
   b. independent
   c. dependent
   d. nominal

5. The research nurse is coding adults according to size. A person with a below-average body mass index (BMI) is coded as 1, average is 2, and above average is 3. What level of measurement is this?
   a. nominal
   b. ratio
   c. ordinal
   d. interval

6. You are asked to design a study measuring how nutritional status is related to serum lead levels in children. You assess calcium and fat intake, as well as serum lead levels in a sample of 30 children who are 2 years old. Lead levels are measured in micrograms per deciliter (mcg/dL). One child had a lead level of 17 mcg/dL. This is an example of what type of variable?

    a. quantitative
    b. qualitative
    c. independent
    d. nominal

Questions 7–9: You are asked to design a study to examine the relationship between preoperative blood pressure and postoperative hematocrit.

7. What is your independent variable?

8. What is your dependent variable?

9. How will you measure each, and what level of measurement is this?

Questions 10–13: You are later asked to do a follow-up study to see whether requiring an intraoperative blood transfusion had an impact on postoperative rates of poor mental health, specifically depression.

10. What is your independent variable?

11. What is your dependent variable?

12. How will you measure these variables, and why?

13. Is your dependent variable measured at the highest level? If not, why not?

Questions 14–18: You decide to measure depression on the following scale: 1 = low, 2 = moderate, 3 = high.

14. What level of measurement is this?

15. How could this measure be improved?

16. Why might you want to improve it?

17. You decide to measure postoperative hematocrit by serum levels. Is this a quantitative or qualitative measurement?

18. You discover that all but those with the lowest hematocrits had higher levels of depression after their surgery and transfusion. Why might the group that had the most critical need for the transfusions not have the subsequent depression associated with this result in the rest of your sample?

Questions 19–25: Elevated serum lead levels in childhood are associated with lower IQ, hyperactivity, aggression, poor growth, diminished academic performance, increased delinquency, seizures, and even death. The neurological damage that occurs cannot be reversed, even once exposure is stopped.

19. You have been asked to follow up in your community and determine what outcomes are associated with lead exposure in children. List three dependent variables for your study and how you will measure them.

20. What level of measurement are your dependent variables? Are they continuous or categorical?

21. Can you increase the level of measurement for any of them?

22. If you are looking at what outcomes are associated with lead exposure in children, what is your independent variable?

23. Why might this independent variable be difficult to measure?

24. Describe how this independent variable could be measured quantitatively or qualitatively.

25. Which way do you prefer to measure the independent variable? Why?

Questions 26–34: A nurse researcher is assessing how well patients respond to two different dosing regimens of a new drug approved to treat diabetic neuropathy. Two different dosing regimens are administered, and side effects are monitored. Results are shown in **Table 1-2**.

TABLE 1-2	Self-Reported Side Effects of Two Randomized Groups of 100 Individuals Treated for Diabetic Neuropathy	
Side Effect Reported	**Low Dosage**	**High Dosage**
Nausea	8	21
Headache	3	5
Weight gain	1	0
Weight loss	0	6
Lethargy	3	11
Skin rash	13	13

26. What is the independent variable?

27. What is the dependent variable?

28. In this study, the nurse researcher measures the side effects as present or not present. This variable is what level of measurement?

29. If instead the nurse researcher decided to measure weight gain in pounds, what level of measurement would it be? Would it be a continuous or categorical variable?

30. If the nurse researcher decided to measure nausea as present, limiting, or debilitating, what level of measurement would it be? Would nausea be a continuous or categorical variable?

31. If the nurse researcher measured nausea as the number of hours of nausea experienced in a day, what level of measurement would it be?

32. If the nurse researcher asked the subjects to describe their headache, would this be a quantitative or a qualitative variable?
In the second phase of this study, the nurse researcher asks the study participants to report changes in signs and symptoms of their neuropathy. She determines that those on the low-dose regimen had a similar level of pain relief and improvement in mobility as those who took the high-dose drug regimen.

33. What is the dependent variable in the second phase of the study?

34. Considering the information you now know about the side effects and relief of neuropathy symptoms, what might you prefer as a patient? Why? What else might you want to know before making the decision?

Questions 35–38: Relate to the following content.

35. You complete a study in which you categorize the subject's blood pressure as normal, prehypertensive, high blood pressure stage 1, or high blood pressure stage 2 using the following criteria. What level of measurement is the stage of high blood pressure?
36. You are now interested in examining compliance with a DASH diet. You ask your subjects if they have or have not complied with the diet this week. Your dietary compliance variable is what level of measurement?
37. After meeting with your statistician, you measure compliance with the DASH diet on a scale of 1 to 7. For analysis purposes, the dietary compliance variable is now what level of measurement? Why might the statistician have recommended this change?
38. You conclude your study by examining how compliance with the DASH diet affects the stage of high blood pressure. What is your independent variable?
39. What is your dependent variable? Is it continuous or categorical?

Statistics: Is what you observe what you expected?

ANSWERS TO ODD-NUMBERED CHAPTER 1 REVIEW QUESTIONS

1. d

3. a

5. c

7. Preoperative blood pressure

9. Answers will vary: actual blood pressure ratio, lab-reported hematocrit ratio, and so on.

11. Depression

13. Answers will vary.

15. Use of interval data, such as Beck's depression scale

17. Quantitative

19. Answers will vary: including IQ, school enrollment, crime, pregnancy, hematocrit, learning disabilities, growth, hearing, and behavior.

21. Answers will vary.

23. Answers will vary: including "It requires a blood draw," "There are different testing mechanisms," "The level may change depending on when the exposure occurred and the time that has lapsed since then," "Levels may differ from fingersticks versus serum draws."

25. Answers will vary.

27. Side effects, nausea, headache, weight gain, weight loss, lethargy, skin rash

29. Ratio, continuous

31. Ratio

33. Signs and symptoms of neuropathy

35. Ordinal

37. Interval; because collecting the data at a higher level of measurement gives you more analysis options

39. Stage of high blood pressure, categorical

CHAPTER 2

PRESENTING DATA

WILL MY AUDIENCE BE ABLE TO SEE WHAT THE DATA IS SAYING?

OBJECTIVES

By the end of this chapter students will be able to:

- Describe a frequency distribution.
- Calculate the cumulative frequency and the cumulative percentages for a group of data.
- Identify situations in which a grouped frequency distribution is helpful.

- Develop a frequency distribution.
- Calculate a percentage.
- Identify the best visual representation for various types of data.
- Determine the percentile rank of an observation.

KEY TERMS

Bar chart
A chart that has the nominal variable on the horizontal axis and the frequency of the response on the vertical axis, with spaces between the bars on the horizontal axis.

Box and whisker plot
A diagram of the central value and variability seen in a data set, with a box containing the median and middle two quartiles of a data set and lines extending out to form "whiskers," which represent the first and fourth quartiles of a data set.

Cumulative frequency
The number of observations with a value less than the maximum value of the variable interval.

Cumulative percentage
The percentage of observations with a value less than the maximum value of the variable interval.

Cumulative relative frequency
A number calculated by adding together all the relative frequencies less than or equal to the selected upper limit point.

Frequency distribution
A summary of the numerical counts of the values or categories of a measurement.

Grouped frequency
A frequency distribution with distinct intervals or groups created to simplify the information.

Histogram
A chart that usually has an ordinal variable on the horizontal axis and the frequency of the response on the vertical axis, with no spaces between the columns on the horizontal axis.

Line graph
A chart in which the horizontal axis shows the passage of time and the vertical axis marks the value of the variable at that particular time.

Outlier
An extreme value of a variable, one that is outside the expected range.

Percentage
A portion of the whole.

Percentile rank
The percentage of observations below a particular value.

Percentiles
One hundred equal portions of a data set.

Quartiles
Four equal portions of a data set, with the first quartile being the 25th percentile, the second quartile being the 50th percentile, and the third quartile being the 75th percentile.

Relative frequency
The number of times a particular observation occurs divided by the total number of observations.

Scatterplot
A chart in which each point represents the measurement of one subject in terms of two variables.

FREQUENCY DISTRIBUTIONS

Once you have designed a study and collected data, the next step is to decide how to present the assembled data. You have several options for doing so. The first and most common choice is a **frequency distribution**, which shows the frequency of each measure of a variable. A frequency distribution is created by gathering all the responses collected from a sample of variables into a table like the one in **Table 2-1**. The first column of the frequency distribution in the table shows the number of days spent postoperatively in the hospital (the dependent variable), sorted from the shortest stay to the longest. The second column shows how frequently that length of stay was needed, that is, the number of patients who spent each number of postoperative days in the hospital. These two columns display the total numeric value of the variable of interest (in this case, the dependent variable, days spent in the hospital),

usually ordered from the lowest to the highest. You can see the frequency of each level of the variable and its spread (distribution).

Sometimes it is also helpful to include the **relative frequency** of an observation, which is just the number of times a particular observation occurs divided by the total number of observations. For example, according to Table 2-1, seven patients stayed in the hospital for 3 days. If you want to report the relative frequency of staying 3 days, divide the number of patients who stayed for 3 days by the total number of patients included in the study; in this example that would be 7 divided by 50, or a relative frequency of 14%. Relative frequency is a helpful concept to illustrate what proportion of the observations this particular observation is. The frequency distribution table presents a big-picture view of your data.

To augment a frequency distribution table and really impress your colleagues, you can add a **cumulative frequency** column, which simply lists the number of observations with a value less than the maximum value of the variable interval. For example, in the third column of Table 2-1, in the second row, the number 9 means that nine patients have stayed either 0, 1, 2, or 3 days postop in the hospital. The number 9 is the cumulative frequency for the first four intervals (0, 1, 2, and 3 days) of the variable. Let's say you are putting together an in-service presentation and decide to collect data from a set of patients on how many postop days they spent in the hospital. You find that nine patients were discharged on day 3 or earlier; that total includes all the patients who stayed for 0, 1, 2, or 3 days. It is a cumulative frequency. You may also want to report a **cumulative relative frequency**, which totals the relative frequencies up to the upper limit point you have selected.

TABLE 2-1	**Frequency Distribution Table for the Length of the Hospital Stay**	
Days Spent in the Hospital Postop	**Number of Patients Who Stayed This Long (Frequency)**	**Number of Patients Who Stayed This Long or Less (Cumulative Frequency)**
0	0	0
1	0	0
2	2	2
3	7	9
4	23	32
5	14	46
6	4	50

In this example, if you wanted to report the cumulative relative frequency for staying 3 days or less, you would simply add the relative frequencies for those staying 0, 1, 2, and 3 days (0/50 + 0/50 + 2/50 + 7/50 = 9/50, or 0.18, or 18%). This can be helpful when presenting your report because most individuals can understand percentages fairly well.

Now your nurse manager approaches you in a panic because the accreditation agency is coming next week, and she needs to know how many patients were discharged after more than 4 days of recovery. The best way to answer that question visually is to create a new table that includes **grouped frequencies**, which are frequency distributions with distinct intervals or groups created to simplify the information. In **Table 2-2**, the values of the frequency distribution in Table 2-1 have been collected into two groups: (1) patients who spent 4 days or fewer in postop and (2) those who spent 5 days or more. Grouped frequencies are typically used when working with a lot of data and an entire frequency distribution is simply too large to be meaningful.

Unfortunately, when data is grouped, some information is lost. For example, how many patients in Table 2-2 stayed for only 2 days? The answer is not discernible from this table.

This is the first drawback to be aware of when using grouped frequencies; you can lose a lot of information when you convert your data into groups, especially if you use large intervals. You can even make the intervals so large that they are meaningless. In our example, if one interval were more than 7 days and the other were less than 7 days, Table 2-2 would not be very useful anymore because all the patients in the study were discharged by day 7. On the other hand, make sure not to make the intervals too small, or your grouped frequency won't have any benefit over a standard frequency distribution.

Let's return to our example of the poor nurse manager who needed to get ready for the accreditation agency visit. After retabulating the data as shown in Table 2-2, you can calmly tell her that during the period of time in your study, 18 patients were discharged after more than 4 days of recovery.

PERCENTAGES

A **percentage** is a part of the whole. To calculate a percentage, divide the partial number of items by the total number of items, and then multiply that quantity by 100. For example, what if that same nurse manager asked you, "What percentage of our patients do those 18 represent?" You could do the simple calculation shown in **Figure 2-1**. In

TABLE 2-2	Frequency Distribution Table for the Length of Hospital Stay Using Grouped Frequencies
Days Spent in the Hospital Postop	**Number of Patients Who Stayed This Long (Frequency)**
≤ 4 days	32
5 or more days	18

FIGURE 2-1	Calculating a Percentage.

$$\frac{18}{50} = 0.36 \times 100 = 36\%$$

TABLE 2-3	Cumulative Percentage Table for Length of Hospital Stay		
Days Spent in the Hospital Postop	**Number of Patients Who Stayed This Long**	**Cumulative Frequency**	**Cumulative Percentage**
0	0	0	$0/50 = 0 \times 100 = 0\%$
1	0	0	$0/50 = 0 \times 100 = 0\%$
2	2	2	$2/50 = 0.04 \times 100 = 4\%$
3	7	9	$9/50 = 0.18 \times 100 = 18\%$
4	23	32	$32/50 = 0.64 \times 100 = 64\%$
5	14	46	$46/50 = 0.92 \times 100 = 92\%$
6	4	50	$50/50 = 1.0 \times 100 = 100\%$

this example, the number of patients of interest (those who were discharged after day 4) is 18. The total number of patients studied is 50. (See the last line of the third column in Table 2-1.) The first step in our calculation is 18 divided by 50. This division results in 0.36, which is then multiplied by 100 to get a percentage of 36%.

Exam scores are a classic example of percentages. If you take an exam with 30 questions and get 27 correct, what is your overall score? In this case, divide 27 by 30, and then multiply by 100 to get 90%.

A statistics concept commonly associated with percentages is **cumulative percentage**, which is the percentage of observations with a value less than the maximum value of the variable interval. The idea is the same as cumulative frequency, but it is expressed as a percentage. The last column in **Table 2-3** shows the conversion of each cumulative frequency (from Table 2-1) into a cumulative percentage: the percentage of patients who had a hospital stay of less than or equal to the number of days listed in that row. For example, 18% of patients had a hospital stay of less than or equal to 3 days,

and all of the patients (100%) were discharged on or before day 6 (see the last line of the last column in the table).

Percentages are also closely related to percentiles, which are explained in the next "From the Statistician."

Percentages are also related to the concept of the **percentile rank** of a score, which is the percentage of observations lower than that score in a frequency distribution. For example, if your test score is greater than 75% of all the scores for the class, it is at the 75th percentile.

BAR CHARTS

Remember nominal categorical data (the categorical data that shows only a difference and is not rank-ordered)? A **bar chart** is one way to display this type of data. A common way to set up the bar chart is to line up the responses for the nominal variable along the horizontal axis and place the frequencies of the responses on the vertical axis. Bar charts are typically used for nominal categorical data with spaces between the bars because

FROM THE STATISTICIAN *Brendan Heavey*

Quantiles, Quartiles, and Percentiles—Oh My!

The terms *quantiles*, *quartiles*, and *percentiles* cause a lot of grief because they are so closely related. So let's break them down a little. Using quantiles is just like dividing a data set into different portions or bins. Two special cases of quantiles are percentiles and quartiles.

- **Percentiles** divide a data set into 100 equal portions. You see this concept used with body mass index (BMI). If a patient's BMI is in the 90th percentile, then 90% of the BMIs in the reference population used to develop the distribution were at or below this patient's BMI. Put another way, this patient's BMI is in the top 10% of the reference population.
- **Quartiles** divide a data set into four equal parts. For example, suppose your nursing manager wants to hire only students who finished in the top quarter of the class on a particular exam. She would calculate the third quartile and select all the scores above it. Because your score would clearly be near the top, she would then rush to your school and attempt to woo you with new scrubs and tuition benefits!

How would the nursing manager compute a percentile? Let's say a sample of 331 nurses at Massachusetts General Hospital is asked how many patients they see on average each shift. The results of this survey are shown in **Table 2-4**. A nice formula to find percentiles in the ordered data set is shown in **Figure 2-2**. For instance, based on the ordered data set in Table 2-4, we apply the formula as shown in Figure 2-2 to find what is called the median, or the middle observation when the observations are lined up in rank order (least to greatest). The median is also the 50th percentile. Therefore, our median is our 166th observation. Using **Figure 2-3**, we can see that the nurse who was observation number 166 saw 16 patients.

Because the total sample is 331, the middle observation is the 166th observation. If you add all the nurses who saw fewer than 16 patients, you find that 155 of them reported seeing fewer than 16 patients, and 22 others saw 16 patients. After lining up the observations in rank order, the 166th observation falls into the group who reported seeing 16 patients; that group is the median. Using the formula takes less time than the old-fashioned way: adding them up.

You can also check yourself by looking at the cumulative relative frequency column. The median should be where the midpoint is. In Table 2-4, look at the row for 15 patients, and see the corresponding cumulative frequency percentage; 47% of the nurses reported seeing 15 or fewer patients. Look at the next line, for 16 patients; 53% of the nurses reported seeing 16 or fewer patients. Therefore, the 50th percentile is above 15 and less than or equal to 16. Because we cannot split a patient into parts (at least for statistical purposes!), the median number of patients is 16.

TABLE 2-4	**Frequency Table for a Sample of 331 Nurses at Massachusetts General Hospital**

Number of Patients	Number of Nurses	Relative Frequency (%)	Cumulative Relative Frequency (%)	Number of Patients	Number of Nurses	Relative Frequency (%)	Cumulative Relative Frequency (%)
1	0	0	0	16	22	7	53
2	0	0	0	17	20	6	60
3	2	1	1	18	19	6	65
4	3	1	2	19	18	5	71
5	5	2	3	20	19	6	76
6	8	2	5	21	17	5	82
7	8	2	8	22	15	5	86
8	9	3	11	23	12	4	90
9	9	3	13	24	8	2	92
10	12	4	17	25	9	3	95
11	14	4	21	26	5	2	96
12	18	5	27	27	5	2	98
13	22	7	33	28	3	1	99
14	23	7	40	29	3	1	100
15	22	7	47	30	1	0	100

Three hundred and thirty-one nurses at Massachusetts General Hospital were asked how many patients they saw on their shifts that night. Relative frequencies are computed by dividing the number of nurses who saw each number of patients by the total number of nurses (331). Each cumulative relative frequency is the result of adding the previous row's relative frequency to its cumulative relative frequency, so in essence, cumulative relative frequency is an accumulation of relative frequency.

(continues)

FROM THE STATISTICIAN *Brendan Heavey*

| FIGURE 2-2 | **Formula for Calculating Percentiles in an Ordered Data Set.** |

$$P_{obs}^{th} = (n+1) \times \frac{y}{100}$$

Where

$P_{obs}^{th} =$ The number of the observations at the percentile for which you are looking

$n =$ The number of observations in your data set

$y =$ The percentile you're looking for

| FIGURE 2-3 | **Equation for the Massachusetts General Sample.** |

$$P_{obs}^{th} = (331+1) \times \frac{50}{100} = 166$$

each answer is distinct and in no particular order. For example, if you collected data about the marital status of fellow nurses on your unit, you might find the data shown in **Figure 2-4**. A quick look at the bar chart makes it apparent that more of the nurses working on this unit are single than either married or other. The bar chart gives you a good visual representation of nominal categorical data.

Figure 2-5 shows another example of a bar chart that represents the data we first examined

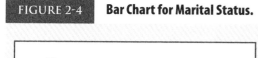

FIGURE 2-4   **Bar Chart for Marital Status.**

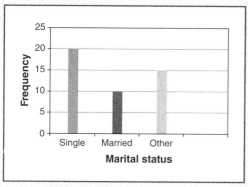

in Chapter 1 about population projections in various states for our public health study. By glancing at the bar chart, we can quickly determine that the population in the state of Florida is substantially larger than the population in Kansas.

Bar charts can be used for ordinal data as well, but then the bars should follow the rank order of the variable categories. For example, if you are presenting the data in **Figure 2-6** about pain levels post hysterectomy at a conference and a listener reports that the policy at his institution is to prescribe pain medication for

FIGURE 2-5   **Projected Populations by State, 2004–2030.**

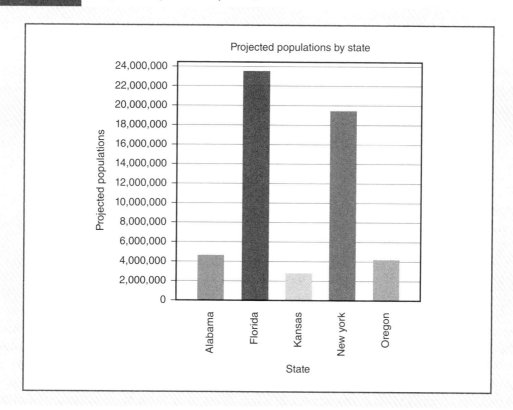

Data from CDC. Population Projections, United States, 2004–2030, by state, age, sex, on CDC WONDER Online Database, September 2005. Retrieved from http://wonder.cdc.gov/population-projections.html.

FIGURE 2-6 **Pain Level 2 Weeks Post Hysterectomy.**

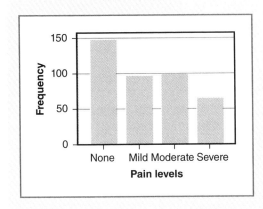

FIGURE 2-7 **How Often Do Subjects Eat Each Day.**

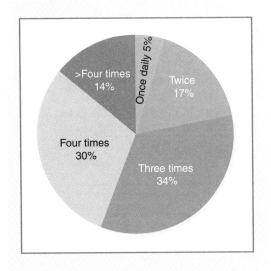

2 weeks upon discharge because patients are fully recovered at that point, your bar chart might be very helpful. You would be able to show quickly that, in your study, the majority of patients are pain-free or close to it (mild pain) by 2 weeks post hysterectomy, but there are still a substantial number who have moderate to severe pain 2 weeks after their procedure. Because the pain variable is measured at an ordinal level, it is useful to have it in rank order on the x axis to illustrate the subsequent escalation of the pain level reported.

Another option for displaying nominal data is a pie chart. In this type of graph, a large circle (the pie) is divided into smaller pieces, and each piece illustrates a percentage of the whole. If you are conducting a study about dietary habits and had a survey question that asks about the frequency of eating each day, you might choose to illustrate the data with the pie chart in **Figure 2-7**. Again, it is easy to see that the majority of your subjects eat 3 to 4 times a day.

HISTOGRAMS

A **histogram** is a type of bar chart. Histograms often have no spaces between the bars because these charts are most frequently used to display either ordinal data or continuous data. (Remember, ordinal data has categories that show a ranked difference; continuous data has an infinite number of possible, in-between measures.) In our previous example, pain may be rated as mild, moderate, or severe. Instead of developing a bar chart and putting the ordinal pain data in rank order on the x axis, we might want to put those bars right next to each other in a histogram. The lack of spaces between the bars in the histogram reinforces the idea that these responses are on a continuum and that the order is illustrated on that continuum.

Presenting these types of data in a histogram shows how frequently each response is

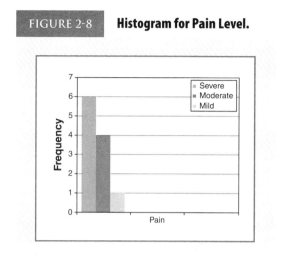

FIGURE 2-8   **Histogram for Pain Level.**

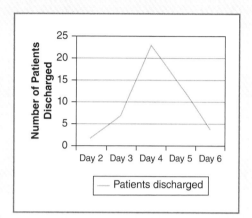

FIGURE 2-9   **Line Graph for Length of Hospitalization.**

selected and allows for visual comparison of the different levels. In **Figure 2-8**, 11 patients were interviewed 12 hours after abdominal surgery. Six rated their pain as severe, four stated it was moderate, and one felt it was only mild (she had just had her pain meds).

This histogram gives you a big-picture idea of the pain these patients experienced. In this case, the histogram seems to indicate that many postop patients report the first 24 hours as being very painful. So the next time you orient a new nurse, you might remember to point out how important it is to make sure patients have their pain medicine ordered and administered immediately after surgery. The chart also visually displays that many patients may not be getting adequate pain medication because so many report severe pain. After collecting this data, you may decide to review the unit protocols for pain management.

LINE GRAPHS

Continuous variables that change over time are frequently best illustrated in a **line graph**.

The horizontal axis shows the passage of time, and the vertical axis marks the value of the variable over time. For example, the data from the cumulative frequency example about days of hospitalization is illustrated in **Figure 2-9**. The chart shows that most of the patients needed to stay 4 days postop before going home. You might want to compare this line graph to another after you institute an early mobilization plan with your surgical patients to see whether the length of hospitalization has changed.

SCATTERPLOTS

Scatterplots are a little different from the previously discussed graphs in that each point represents how one subject relates to two variables. For example, **Figure 2-10** shows a scatterplot of height in inches and weight in pounds for a group of eight kindergartners. Each square on the scatterplot represents one student. The horizontal axis displays that student's height,

FIGURE 2-10   **Scatterplot for Student Height (*x* axis) and Weight (*y* axis).**

and the vertical axis displays his or her weight. You can see from the direction of the plotted points that as students get taller, they usually get heavier as well; that's the relationship between the two variables. When points are close together or seem to follow a line closely, the relationship between the variables on the horizontal and vertical axes are relatively strong.

When you look at a scatterplot, note the general trend. In this example, the plotted points start low on the left side and move up as they progress toward the right side. This pattern indicates a *positive relationship* between height and weight (in other words, they usually move in the same direction—when height increases, weight usually does too). If the plotted points were to start in the upper left corner and slope down to the right, the pattern would indicate a *negative relationship* between the two variables (such as exercise and weight—when exercise is increased, weight usually decreases).

Scatterplots also give nurses a chance to look for **outliers**, or data that is outside the expected

relationship. In Figure 2-10, the student who is only 30 inches and 20 pounds clearly stands out from the rest of the group. Perhaps the child is just extremely small, or there may have been an error in measurement, recording, or data entry. If there are a many outliers, a nurse may decide either that further investigation is needed to ensure accuracy or that the outliers may actually represent the children whom the study is designed to identify. One example of this technique is the use of growth charts. When children make pediatric visits, nurses almost always plot the children's heights and weights on a growth chart. This is one example of using a scatterplot to look for outliers. If a child isn't growing properly, recognizing the growth pattern as an outlier is one way to identify a child who needs intervention.

BOX AND WHISKERS PLOT

Sometimes when we want to find outliers, or we want to illustrate the central value and variability seen in a data set, we may opt to use a diagram called a **box and whiskers plot** (see **Figure 2-11**). In this type of diagram, the observations are lined up from least to most, and the quartiles (first 25% of observations, second 25% of observations, third 25% of observations, and fourth 25% of observations) are identified. The middle 50% (quartile 2 and 3) of the data set is contained in the box of the diagram, and the whiskers of the diagram show the range of the data. Notice that there is an observation at a value of 2, which is not contained in the range of the whiskers. Individual dots at the far end of a box and whiskers plot are considered outliers. We will talk about this in more detail in the next chapter when we start to look at measures of central tendency.

| FIGURE 2-11 | **Box and Whiskers Plot.** |

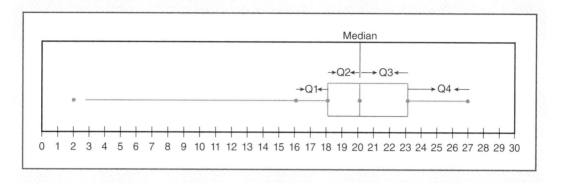

SUMMARY

This chapter contained quite a bit of information, so let's review and make sure you are really comfortable with it. Frequently, researchers put a great deal of time into collecting data and very little time into thinking about how to present it; however, how you present your data often determines whether your intended audience understands your work or is even interested in it. (Teachers are all aware of this point!) The most common choice for presentations is a frequency distribution, which shows the frequency of each measure of a variable. You can add these frequencies and create either cumulative frequency columns or grouped frequencies, depending on the question you are trying to answer.

You can also calculate percentages, which are parts of the whole. Because many nurses are familiar with them, percentages are sometimes a useful way to convey information. You can then add the percentages and present a cumulative percentage, which is simply the percentage of observations with a value less than the maximum value of the interval.

Another way to convey information is with a visual graph, such as a bar chart for nominal data, a histogram for ordinal or continuous data, a line graph for continuous variables that change over time, or a scatterplot in which one subject's values for two variables are graphed. You need to decide which type of chart will work the best for the audience you are trying to reach. Just remember, use color, make it bigger, and avoid using lots and lots of numbers in a row—and bring coffee because most nurses are considerably sleep deprived!

CHAPTER 2 REVIEW QUESTIONS

1. Thirty fathers were asked about the highest level of education they had completed. Ten completed only elementary school, 10 completed elementary and high school, 7 completed all levels through college, and 3 completed all levels through graduate school. What was the cumulative percentage of fathers who completed only elementary school? Round to the nearest whole number.

2. In your study of 40 people, 8 had no cold symptoms, 12 had mild cold symptoms, 9 had moderate cold symptoms, and 10 had severe cold symptoms. One patient was lost to follow-up, and no data could be collected. What percentage of patients reported cold symptoms?

3. Given the information in review question 2, what percentage of patients reported no cold symptoms?

4. Use the frequency distribution in **Table 2-5** to construct a bar chart for influenza cases in your hospital during 8 months in 2017-2018. Would your chart look different if it were a histogram? Discuss at least one rationale for selecting either a bar chart or a histogram to present this data.

Questions 5–7: Your community begins a large-scale influenza vaccine effort, and the following year, the number of cases drops (see **Table 2-6**).

5. Construct a line graph showing the data from 2017 and the data from 2018. Compare the two.

6. Why didn't the numbers change significantly for August and September?

7. Do you consider the vaccine effort to be successful? Why?

TABLE 2-5	Influenza Cases for 2017
Month	**Number of Cases**
August	18
September	29
October	68
November	107
December	158
January	166
February	160
March	111

TABLE 2-6	Influenza Cases for 2018
Month	**Number of Cases**
August	19
September	27
October	31
November	34
December	48
January	59
February	51
March	45

Research Application

Questions 8–13: See the data in **Table 2-7**.

8. Construct a bar chart for mother's marital status.

TABLE 2-7	**Demographic Characteristics of 92 Adolescents Completing a Family Planning Survey**

	n (%)
Pregnancy status	
Pregnant	78 (84.7)
Not pregnant	14 (15.2)
Age	
≤ 14 years old	2 (2.2)
15–17 years old	46 (50)
18–19 years old	43 (46.7)
*Number in household**	
< 6 people	70 (79.5)
≥ 6 people	18 (20.5)
Student status[†]	
Not in school	46 (50.5)
In school	45 (49.4)
Mother's marital status	
Single	38 (41.3)
Married	27 (29.3)
Divorced	13 (14.1)
Other	14 (15.2)
Employment status	
Employed	25 (27.2)
Not employed	67 (72.8)

*Missing *n* = 4
[†]Missing *n* = 1
Reproduced from Heavey, E. Moysich, K., Hyland, A., Druschel, C., & Sill, M. (2008) Female adolescents' perceptions of male partners' pregnancy desire. *Journal of Midwifery & Women's Health, 53*(4), 338-344. Reproduced with permission of Elsevier Inc.

9. What percentage of the adolescents are employed? What percentage of the adolescents are in school? Are these variables quantitative or qualitative? Round to the nearest tenth of a percent.

10. Identify the level of measurement of each variable.

11. Could any of these variables have been measured as continuous quantitative variables?

12. Construct a histogram for the ages of the adolescents. Describe the histogram and what it tells you about this sample population. Why would a histogram be an appropriate choice for presenting this data?

13. Is the pregnancy status of this group of adolescents typical? Why might that be?

14. You've been recruited by the head of the Federal Emergency Management Agency (FEMA) to act as the head triage nurse for a large city's hurricane response team. One of your main duties is to decide which nurses will cover which facilities in the overall relief effort. Because most nursing duties will have to change during this shift in personnel, you decide to divide the group based on years of experience. Your nurse's aide carries out a brief survey of all the personnel available (100 nurses) and gives you a list of the number of years of experience for each (see **Table 2-8**). Find the quartiles of this distribution, and assign a role to each nurse. For example, the nurses with the least amount of experience should be assigned to the rescue team, and the ones with the most experience should be assigned to the intensive care unit (ICU).

Questions 15–18: A diabetes educator is working with a group of 15 patients who have been newly diagnosed with type 2 diabetes. She administers a brief pretest, reviews carbohydrate counting with them, and then asks them to complete a posttest assessing their knowledge of the total grams of carbohydrate found in one serving of four sample items brought to the class. The results are shown in **Table 2-9**.

15. Complete the Cumulative Frequency column of the table.

16. What percentage of the patients answered all four questions correctly?

TABLE 2-8	**Nurses Available for the Hurricane Response Team**		
Number of Years' Experience	**Number of Nurses**	**Number of Years' Experience**	**Number of Nurses**
2	15	12	3
3	10	13	3
4	9	15	3
5	8	18	3
6	8	20	2
7	9	25	2
8	6	32	1
9	5	35	1
10	5	36	1
11	5	40	1

	Coordinated Hurricane Response		
Rescue Team	Stadium	Hospital	ICU

TABLE 2-9	**Posttest Assessing Carbohydrate Knowledge**	
Number Correct on the Posttest	**Number of Patients Who Answered This Number of Questions Correctly (Frequency)**	**Number Who Answered This Many or Fewer Questions Correctly (Cumulative Frequency)**
0	1	
1	1	
2	2	
3	6	
4	5	

17. Add another column to the table, and calculate the cumulative percentage.

18. The diabetes educator would like you to present her results in a grouped frequency table showing the frequency and percentage of those who passed the posttest with >70% and those who didn't for the report she has to make to her funding agency. Show your product.

Questions 19–20: A researcher examining patients diagnosed with sarcoidosis would like to look at trends in their inflammatory markers. The researcher would like to use a graph that can illustrate the erythrocyte sedimentation rate and the C-reactive protein level for each individual in the study and thus show the relationship between the two markers.

19. What graphic representation of the data would you suggest?

20. After creating this graph, the researcher notices one of the subjects is significantly below the trend line that the other subjects seem to follow. What might be a logical explanation for this outlier?

21. An emergency room nurse working in a hospital in the wine region of the Finger Lakes in New York has noticed a seasonal trend for ocular injuries from bottle corks. She would like to illustrate this graphically and develops a histogram. Why might she prefer a histogram to a bar chart?

22. When the nurse looks at her data and the histogram, it is apparent that more ocular injuries from bottle corks occur in October (which is wine fermentation season) and January. She also notices that more of the injuries involve the right eye. Provide a reasonable explanation for both the January peak and the prevalence of the right-eye injuries.

23. The nurse would like to determine if more ocular injuries are associated with wine bottles from Sharespeak Winery or with wine bottles from Francesco's winery. What would be the independent variable?

24. What would be the dependent variable in review question 23?

25. You are tracking melanoma in your county. Calculate the race- and gender-specific mortality rates from the data provided in **Table 2-10.**

TABLE 2-10	**Melanoma Data**			
	New Cases	**Deaths**	**Population**	**Mortality Rate**
Men	5	2	25,000	
Women	3	1	25,000	
White	7	3	40,000	
African American	1	0	10,000	

26. Offer a potential explanation for why the race-specific rates may be different for whites and African Americans.

27. Complete the following table:

Age Range	Number of Subjects in Sample	Cumulative Frequency
0–5	1	
6–10	2	3
11–15		7
16–20	1	8
21–25		11
26–30	4	
31–35	6	

Questions 28–29: The Centers for Disease Control and Prevention (CDC) provided **Table 2-11** and **Figure 2-12** showing mortality rate data from Delaware and California in 2014.

TABLE 2-11

State	Deaths	Population	Rate per 100,000
California	3,539,688	540,469,946	654.9
Delaware	110,279	12,809,756	860.9
Total	3,649,967	553,279,702	659.7

FIGURE 2-12   **Mortality Rates per 100,000 People in California and Delaware in 2014.**

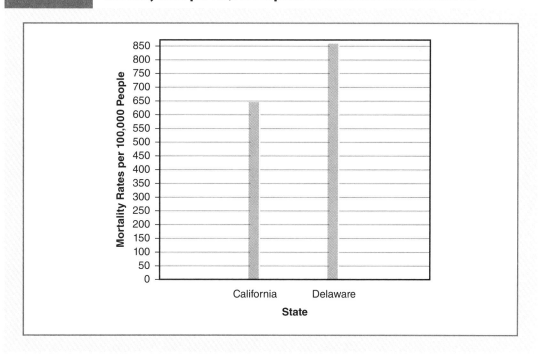

Reproduced from Centers for Disease Control and Prevention, National Center for Health Statistics. Compressed Mortality File 1999-2013. Archive on CDC WONDER Online Database, released October 2014. Data are from the Compressed Mortality File 1999-2013 Series 20 No. 25, 2014, as compiled from data provided by the 57 vital statistics jurisdictions through the Vital Statistics Cooperative Program. Accessed at http://wonder.cdc.gov/cmf-icd10-archive2013.html on Apr 4, 2017.

28. Your colleague has a pending job offer and decides he will accept the offer in Delaware because too many people die in California every year. Do you agree with his decision? Why or why not?

29. Which is more effective for presenting the data about mortality rates: the table or the bar chart? Why?

30. **Table 2-12** presents data from the CDC that tracks Ebola cases in Sierra Leone in June 2014. Complete the Cumulative Frequency columns.

TABLE 2-12

Date	Number of Cases	Cumulative Frequency, Cases	Number of Deaths	Cumulative Frequency, Deaths
6/2/2014	50		6	
6/5/2014	81		7	
6/10/2014	89		7	
6/11/2014	117		19	
6/18/2014	97		49	
6/24/2014	158		34	

Data from CDC. (2016). *2014 Ebola outbreak in West Africa* — Reported case graphs. Retrieved from https://www.cdc.gov/vhf/ebola/outbreaks/2014-west-africa/cumulative-cases-graphs.html

Questions 31–33: Refer to the graph in **Figure 2-13.**

31. Which age group has the highest incidence of chlamydia? What explanations might the researchers offer about this data?

32. Which group has the lowest incidence of chlamydia? What explanations might the researchers offer about this data?

33. If you were going to design a chlamydia prevention campaign, what age group would you suggest targeting? Why?

FIGURE 2-13   **Incidence of Chlamydia in Florida by Age Group.**

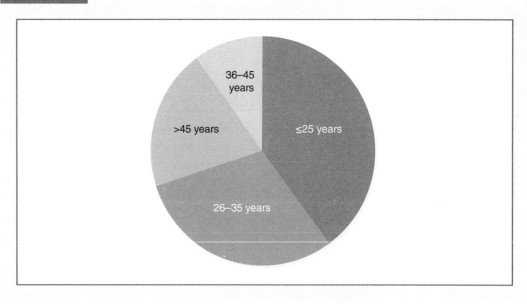

ANSWERS TO ODD-NUMBERED CHAPTER 2 REVIEW QUESTIONS

1. 33%

3. 20%

5. Answer includes line graph; beginning in October, there is a substantial decrease in cases.

7. Yes, there was a substantial decrease in cases beginning in October after the vaccine was administered.

9. 27.2%, 49.4%, qualitative

11. Yes, age, number in household, years in school, years employed

13. No, all the adolescents were waiting for pregnancy or family planning—related services.

15.

Number Correct on the Posttest	Number of Patients Who Answered This Number of Questions Correctly (Frequency)	Number Who Answered This Many or Fewer Questions Correctly (Cumulative Frequency)
0	1	1
1	1	2
2	2	4
3	6	10
4	5	15

17.

% Who Answered This Many or Fewer Questions Correctly (Cumulative %)
1/15 = 6.7%
2/15 = 13.3%
4/15 = 26.7%
10/15 = 66.7%
15/15 = 100%

19. A scatterplot

21. A histogram better illustrates the continuum of time from one month to the next with an order involved.

23. The winery

25.

New Cases	Deaths	Population	Mortality Rate	
Men	5	2	25,000	**0.008%**
Women	3	1	25,000	**0.004%**
White	7	3	40,000	**0.0075%**
African American	1	0	10,000	**0**

27.

Age Range	Frequency	Cumulative Frequency
0–5	1	1
6–10	2	3
11–15	4	7
16–20	1	8
21–25	3	11
26–30	4	15
31–35	6	21

29. Putting the rates rather than the absolute numbers in the bar chart helps to illustrate more clearly the different mortality rates between states that are so vastly different in size.

31. The highest incidence is in those who are ≤ 25 years old. Explanations may vary but may include having more sexual partners, practicing riskier sex, and engaging in more frequent sexual activity for people in this age bracket.

33. Answers will vary but may include ages ≤ 25 because of higher incidence and more long-term risks from early infection. May also include all under age 35 because that captures the two highest-incidence age groups.

DESCRIPTIVE STATISTICS, PROBABILITY, AND MEASURES OF CENTRAL TENDENCY

WHAT DOES THE DATA TELL ME?

OBJECTIVES

By the end of this chapter students will be able to:

- Compare and contrast descriptive statistics and inferential statistics.

- Define, distinguish between, and interpret the mean, median, mode, and standard deviation.

- Identify unimodal, bimodal, and multimodal distributions.

- Determine which measure of central tendency is appropriate in a given data set.

- Calculate and interpret a standard deviation and range for a given data set.

- Explain descriptive results from a given data set using a Statistical Package for the Social Sciences (SPSS) printout.

- Define probability and explain the range of possible probabilities.

- Compare and contrast frequency and probability distributions.

- Contrast positive and negative distribution skews and describe where the outliers are present.

KEY TERMS

Bimodal
Having two values or categories that have the highest occurrence and that are equal frequencies.

Central tendency
An indicator of the center of the data.

Extreme outlier
An outlier in a data set that is more than 3 times the interquartile range either above or below the interquartile range ($\pm 3 \times$ the length of the box above or below the box on a box and whiskers plot).

Frequency distribution
Lists all the possible outcomes of an experiment and tallies the number of times each outcome occurs.

Mean
The sum of the values divided by the total number of observations. It is the most commonly known measure of central tendency but requires interval or ratio data.

Median
For ordinal, interval, and ratio data, the value in the middle when all the measured values are lined up in order from least to most; the 50th percentile value.

Mode
The most frequently occurring value or category in the distribution. When a distribution has only one mode, it is called unimodal.

Multimodal
Having more than two modes.

Normal distribution
A probability distribution in which the mean, median, and mode are equal with a bell-shaped distribution curve.

Probability
The chance that a particular outcome will occur after an event.

p-value
The probability of finding the reported results if the null hypothesis is true.

Probability distribution
The probability of all the possible outcomes of the variable.

Range
The difference between the maximum and minimum values in a distribution.

Sampling distribution
Plots realized frequencies of a statistic versus the range of possible values that statistic can take.

Skewed distribution
An asymmetrical distribution of the values of the variable around the mean, making one tail longer than the other.

Standard deviation
The average distance that the values in a distribution are from the center.

Tukey fences
A cutoff value indicating that an observation is an outlier in a data set because it is more than 1.5 times the interquartile range either above or below the interquartile range (± 1.5 times the length of the box above or below the box on a box and whiskers plot).

Z-score
A measure that indicates how many standard deviations a value is from the mean value.

DESCRIPTIVE STATISTICS: PROPERTIES OF VARIABLES

Once the variables of interest in a study have been defined, nurses and statisticians usually look at a set of so-called descriptive statistics that allows them to get to know more about each variable. A variable can be described in two main ways:

- In terms of its central value or tendency
- In terms of how far away the observations are spread from the variable's center

We will start by defining central tendency.

MEASURES OF CENTRAL TENDENCY

Central tendency is an indicator of the center of the data. Defining the central tendency of a distribution more specifically is not easy, however, because the answer depends on the analysis technique used—which in turn depends on the level of measurement of the data. Let's start by reviewing the levels of measurement.

First, *nominal variables* describe categorical differences, such as gender. The only measure of central tendency for nominal data is the **mode**, which is the most frequently occurring measure in the data. For example, if your sample includes 15 men and 5 women, the mode is the 15 men. If you look at the bar graph in **Figure 3-1**, you can easily identify the mode because it is the highest column. This is an example of a unimodal distribution, where there is only one mode.

If a ZIP code sample includes seven people living in 14617, seven people living in 14619, and six people living in 14621, the two values 14617

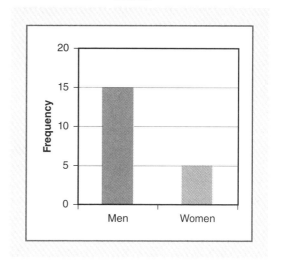

FIGURE 3-1 **Demographic Information: Gender.**

FIGURE 3-2 **Zip Codes Bimodal.**

and 14619 have the highest occurrence and are equal, so the sample has two modes and is called **bimodal**. Again, if you look at a bar chart like the one in **Figure 3-2**, you can easily see that this is a bimodal variable because the two columns for ZIP codes 14617 and 14619 are the same height. Large samples may even be **multimodal**; that is, they have more than two modes.

Data that is rank-ordered (ordinal, interval, or ratio) have a second measure of central tendency: a **median**. If you line up all the measured values in order from least to most, the value in the middle of the list is the median. For example, suppose a set of students has the following scores on their most recent nursing exam: 66, 74, 83, 83, 88, 94, 96, 97, 99. The median score is 88, the one right in the middle. Or suppose that the first person who takes the exam forgets to hand it in, so the number of exams is even: 74, 83, 83, 88, 94, 96, 97, 99. Then the median is actually the average of the fourth and fifth values: (88 + 94) ÷ 2, or 91%.

The mode in this data is 83. You can see that the measures of central tendency do not always produce the same results. This is the main reason why defining central tendency is difficult.

Perhaps the most commonly known measure of central tendency is the **mean**, which is the sum of the values divided by the total number of observations. For example, if you add all the original test scores listed first above and divide by the total number of students who took the test, you find that the mean of the original test scores is 86.67: (66 + 74 + 83 + 83 + 88 + 94 + 96 + 97 + 99 ÷) 9. Again, the mean is not the same as the median or the mode. Each is a different measure of central tendency. They may even be the same number (as in a normal distribution, which we talk about later in this chapter), but they do not have to be and they all have different definitions. The mean can be calculated only if the available data is at the interval or ratio level. You cannot calculate a mean on ordinal or nominal data. Think about it: What is the "average" gender? That question doesn't make sense. Nominal or ordinal data does not lend itself to the calculation of averages. However, even with interval- or ratio-level

data, you may decide to use the median instead of the mean for your measure of central tendency. This is frequently considered the better option.

Why the median is considered a better statistic to use than the mean? Students in any course should be *very* interested in the answer. Let's say the following scores are recorded on a final exam:

32, 35, 38, 40, 41, 41, 42, 43, 44, 45, 46, 47, 48, 99, 100, 100

Clearly, the class, overall, did not do very well on this exam. In fact, of the 16 people who took the exam, only 3 passed, scoring significantly higher than the rest of the class. These three scores are outliers (observations that are significantly different from the rest of the sample) and may distort the mean while leaving the median relatively unaltered. Let's take a look.

- The mean of the data is 52.6
- The median of the data is 43.5.

You can see that the 43.5 is a much better estimate of the central tendency, and in fact the mean is so high only because of the three top scores, which are very different from the rest of the data. If you scored a 48 on this test, you did fairly well in comparison to your classmates, scoring higher than 75% of them. However, what if your professor decided to look just at the mean? She might tell you that you didn't even beat the average grade for the class, even though only three people actually outscored you.

RANGE AND SAMPLE STANDARD DEVIATION

Variables can vary from their center or central tendency, and the variation can be explained by two terms.

- First, the **range** is the difference between the maximum value and minimum value of a variable. For example, in a sample there might be five subjects ages 10, 14, 20, 55, and 95. The age range of the sample is 85 years (95 years minus 10 years), or it can also be reported as 10 to 95 years.

- The **standard deviation** is the average distance of the values from the variable's mean. When the standard deviation is large, the spread among the values in the data set is large, indicating a heterogeneous sample. When the deviation is small, most of the scores are very close to the average score, indicating a more homogeneous sample.

You may find that, although the average heart rate is the same on a postpartum unit as on a cardiac intensive care unit, the ranges and standard deviations in the heart rates are substantially different (see **Figure 3-3**). Postpartum patients are generally a homogenous group of relatively healthy young women with heart rates that should be fairly close to normal. In contrast, cardiac ICU patients are a more heterogeneous sample with a large variation in observed heart rates; some will be quite high and others will be quite low. Both groups may have the same average heart rate, but the ranges and standard deviations in the observed heart rates are substantially different. You can see this idea illustrated graphically in Figure 3-3. The center of the data in each curve is the mean, which is the same in the two samples. However, the observed heart rates in the postpartum sample are distributed tightly around that mean, while the observed heart rates in the cardiac ICU sample are spread out much more.

CALCULATING THE STANDARD DEVIATION

Standard deviation is harder to calculate than range, but not that hard. Suppose you collect heart rates for the patients who are day 1 postdelivery on your postpartum unit and find that the mean heart rate is $(45 + 60 + 75 + 90) \div 4 = 67.5$ (see **Table 3-1**). The formula for the standard deviation (σ) is shown in **Figure 3-4**.

TABLE 3-1	Frequency Table for Heart Rates Day 1 Postpartum
Heart Rate	**Frequency**
45	1
60	1
75	1
90	1

FIGURE 3-3 **Heart Rate.**

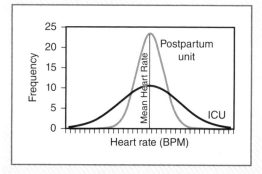

FIGURE 3-4 **Calculating the Sample Standard Deviation.**

$$\sigma = \frac{\sqrt{(x_1 - \mu)^2 + (x_2 - \mu)^2 + (x_n - \mu)^2}}{n-1}$$

Where
x = values in the distribution
μ = mean
σ = Standard deviation

In a less "mathematical" version, it might look like this:

$$\sigma = \sqrt{\frac{(\text{first value} - \text{mean})^2 + (\text{second value} - \text{mean})^2 + \ldots + (n^{\text{th}} - \text{mean})^2}{\text{number of values} - 1}}$$

In our example, then, the standard deviation is the square root of:

$$\frac{(45 - 67.5)^2 + (60 - 67.5)^2 + (75 - 67.5)^2 + (90 - 67.5)^2}{4 - 1}$$

which equals:

$$\frac{(-22.5)(-22.5) + (-7.5)(-7.5) + (7.5)(7.5) + (22.5)(22.5)}{3}$$

or:
$$\frac{506.25 + 56.25 + 56.25 + 506.25}{3}$$

This reduces to what is actually called the sample variance:

$$\frac{1125}{3} = 375$$

FROM THE STATISTICIAN *Brendan Heavey*

Why Is There an $n - 1$ in the Denominator of Sample Variance?

Wouldn't it be a whole lot easier to remember sample variance if the denominator didn't contain an $n - 1$? The answer is yes, remembering the formula would be a heck of a lot easier if we could just scrap the $n - 1$ and throw an n into the denominator. In fact, as the sample size of our data set increases, the $n - 1$ becomes more and more negligible. However, in small samples, we can see that the sample mean is a lot closer to each sample value than the population mean.

Think about it: Although the sample mean is a decent descriptor of the middle of our sample, the population mean doesn't even have to be within the range of our sample! Let's think about an example. If you were interested in estimating the average heart rate of a human being in normal sinus rhythm, you might sample 10 different healthy volunteers. Each volunteer would have small differences in individual heart rate depending on what time of day you took their pulses, how much they had been moving in the moments leading up to your measurement, their body mass index (BMI), and so on. Let's say you chose to test each person's heart rate five different times and took an average of those measurements to report on; your results might look like this:

Heart Rates Measured at Five Different Times

	Person 1	Person 2	Person 3	Person 4	Person 5
	65	65	51	69	79
	62	67	58	72	72
	60	58	55	73	75
	58	62	53	70	78
	61	63	59	76	77
Sample Means	Avg = 61.2	Avg = 63	Avg = 55.2	Avg = 72	Avg = 76.2
Population Mean	Overall Average = 65.52				

FROM THE STATISTICIAN *Brendan Heavey*

Look at how the individual pulse rates vary around their individual sample means. Notice that the overall mean is generally further away from the data points than the sample mean is. In fact, the population mean is not even in the range of Person 5's recorded values. Let's calculate the numerator of Person 5's variance using the sample mean:

$$(79 - 76.2)^2 + (72 - 76.2)^2 + (75 - 76.2)^2 + (78 - 76.2)^2 + (77 - 76.2)^2 = 30.8$$

Now, let's do the same thing but substitute the population mean:

$$(79 - 65.52)^2 + (72 - 65.52)^2 + (75 - 65.52)^2 + (78 - 65.52)^2 + (77 - 65.52)^2 = 601.112$$

Clearly, Person 5 contributes a lot more to the variance component of the population than he or she does to the sample. In general, there is a lot less variance around the sample mean than the population mean, so sample variance tends to underestimate the population variance. You can make up for this difference, or what the statisticians call bias, by putting an $n - 1$ in the denominator of the sample variance calculation.

Then you need to take the square root of 375: 19.36. So the standard deviation in the postpartum sample is 19.36.

I know some of you are starting to wonder, "Why am I in this class again?" Don't get too frustrated by the equations. On the other hand, if you are just dying to know more about variance, read the "From the Statistician" feature, which delves further into this topic. The essential concept to understand is why the standard deviation is important: *It tells you the average distance that the values in your distribution fall from the mean, and it gives you an idea about how much alike or how varied your sample is in terms of the variable you are examining.*

USING A BOX AND WHISKERS PLOT TO DISPLAY CENTRAL TENDENCY AND RANGE

We briefly touched on the box and whiskers plot in the last chapter, but now I suspect some of the terminology involved will make more sense. In the diagram in **Figure 3-5**, you can see a box and whiskers plot that is displayed vertically.

To develop the box and whiskers plot, first line up the strength scores in rank-order, then determine the median and quartiles. The box on each diagram contains the interquartile range (IQR), which is the middle 50% of the strength scores for each gender. The line in the

FIGURE 3-5 **Box and Whiskers Plot: Central Tendency and Range.**

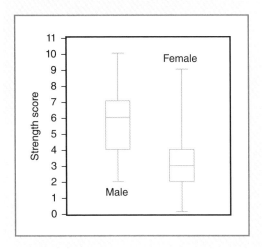

middle of the box is the median strength score for each gender. The "whiskers" illustrate the range of scores seen for each gender. The lower whisker is the first quartile, or the lowest 25% of the observations; the upper whisker is the fourth quartile, or the upper most 25% of the observations. This data set has no identified outliers, which are usually illustrated by an individual dot plotted outside the whiskers. An outlier is frequently defined as a value that is more than 1.5 times the interquartile range (length of the box) either above or below the edges of the box (beginning of quartile 2 and end of quartile 3). These predefined cutoffs used for identifying outliers are referred to as Tukey fences (Tukey, 1977). We can easily tell by looking at the box and whiskers plot that this data set has no identified outliers, the median strength score is higher for men than for women, and women have a greater range of strength scores. This method is a lot faster than looking at the raw data, which is another reason why graphic illustrations can be very helpful when you are presenting your data!

We can also look at a box and whiskers plot horizontally (**Figure 3-6**). No matter what direction the graph is displayed, the concept is the same. It is a visual representation of the center and dispersion of the data set.

FIGURE 3-6 **Box and Whiskers Plot: Horizontal.**

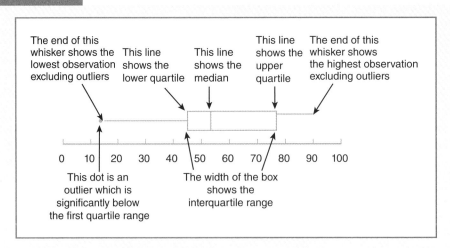

Modified from BBC. (2014). Maths: Statistics and probability. Retrieved from http://www.bbc.co.uk/schools/gcsebitesize/maths/statistics/representingdata3hirev6.shtml

FROM THE STATISTICIAN *Brendan Heavey*

Probability and the Normal Distribution

Probability is a difficult concept to grasp fully. In fact, it has so many different facets that statisticians sometimes have difficulty defining it adequately. The good news is that, at this point, you don't need an in-depth understanding of it. In fact, for the purposes of this text, think of probability as long-run relative frequency. You should know what relative frequency means, but what does "long-run relative frequency" mean? That is an important question, and it doesn't have a very good answer. Let's look at an example to try to explain this concept.

We are going to revisit the age-old experiment of rolling dice. **Table 3-2** shows the results of rolling a single die 10 times and counting how many times the die shows a 3 on its face. The cumulative and relative frequencies associated

TABLE 3-2	**Frequency Table for Rolling a 3 When Rolling a Six-Sided Die**		
Roll	**Result**	**Cumulative Frequency of 3**	**Relative Frequency of 3**
1	1	0	0
2	3	1	$\frac{1}{2} = 0.5$
3	2	1	$\frac{1}{3} = 0.33$
4	5	1	$\frac{1}{4} = 0.25$
5	6	1	$\frac{1}{5} = 0.2$
6	2	1	$\frac{1}{6} = 0.16$
7	3	2	$\frac{1}{7} = 0.29$
8	4	2	$\frac{2}{8} = 0.25$
9	4	2	$\frac{2}{9} = 0.22$
10	6	2	$\frac{2}{10} = 0.2$

(continues)

FROM THE STATISTICIAN *Brendan Heavey*

with each roll are tabulated in the last two columns. This time, we're going to focus on the final column, the relative frequency. The relative frequency is the total number of times you roll a particular value (in this case, 3) out of the total number of rolls.

If you look at the relative frequency column closely, you will notice that it starts out low and then, as soon as we roll a 3, the relative frequency jumps up to 0.5. In fact, if we continued this experiment for a long time, the jumping would continue forever—each time you roll another 3, the numerator increases. However, each jump would be smaller than the last (because each roll also increases the denominator).

Just for fun, we did this very thing and plotted the relative frequency over 1,000 rolls in **Figure 3-7**. Notice that, after a while, the relative frequency of rolling a 3 settles down to around 0.16, or $\frac{1}{6}$. In the beginning, the relative frequency jumps up and down, but after about 100 rolls, we can clearly see the trend settling. We would fully expect this going forward because the die has six sides, and if we rolled the die 1 million times, we would expect somewhere around $\frac{1}{6}$ of the rolls to turn up a 3. Because we can see the main pattern developed after 100 rolls in this experiment, we define "long run" as 100 rolls. Keep in mind, however, that the definition can change between experiments.

FIGURE 3-7   **Graph of the Relative Frequency of Rolling a 3.**

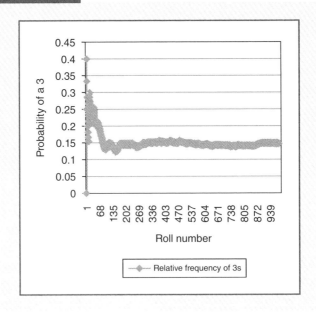

MOVING FORWARD: INFERENTIAL STATISTICS

Once researchers are done describing the variables they are interested in, they usually like to make inferences about populations based on the measurements they have taken in their samples. This practice, called inferential statistics, involves associating probabilities with each variable studied. **Probability** is the chance that a particular outcome will occur. For example, let's say that a class of 100 nursing students has 25 men and 75 women, and we want to know the probability that a randomly chosen student from this class will be female. The answer is 75/100, or 0.75, or 75%. Probabilities are important because, no matter how careful and precise researchers are, there is always some level of uncertainty. Even if the researchers believe the class is composed entirely of men, the researchers cannot say the probability is 1.0, or 100%, that a randomly chosen student will be male; they can only say that the probability approaches 100%. (Did anyone see the Disney movie *Mulan*? A young Chinese woman joins the imperial army disguised as a man. If one were to randomly select an infantry soldier from this "all-male" group, the probability that you would select a man approaches 100%, but there is always room for some error, such as if one were to randomly select Mulan in disguise.) Conversely, the researchers cannot say that the probability of randomly selecting a female from what they believe is an all-male class is 0.0, or 0%. They can only say the probability approaches 0. Probability theory is a science in and of itself, so here we will cover it in a nutshell in the next "From the Statistician" feature.

FREQUENCY DISTRIBUTIONS VERSUS PROBABILITY DISTRIBUTIONS

You may remember that, to create a **frequency distribution**, the researcher lists all the possible outcomes or observations and counts the number of times each outcome occurs. The researcher then graphs these totals to make them easier to visualize and understand. We looked at many examples of how we might choose to display the frequency distribution of our sample data in Chapter 2.

A **probability distribution** graphs the *probability of all the possible outcomes* of the variable "in the long run" instead of their frequency. The sum of all the individual probabilities is 1, or 100%. This also means that the area under the curve in a graphed probability distribution is equal to 1, or 100%. As you can see in the probability distribution in **Figure 3-8**, if we collected the birthweight data of all infants born in our population, the probability of randomly selecting a single infant weighing about seven pounds is about 50%. About half of the birthweight values are below 7 pounds and about half are above. Although frequency distributions and probability distributions look a lot alike, they represent two very distinct concepts.

Probability distributions help us a lot in statistics. For example, as we proceed in the textbook, you will begin running statistical tests to look for associations or differences between variables. Each of these tests is going to produce a *p*-value and (you guessed it) that *p*-value is just the probability of finding the outcome you observed if the null hypothesis is true. (Remember, the null means that there is no relationship or association between the

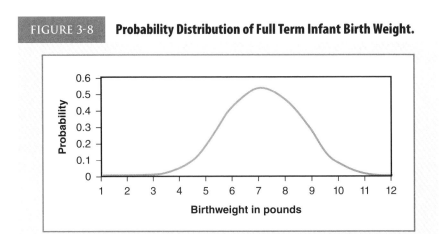

FIGURE 3-8   **Probability Distribution of Full Term Infant Birth Weight.**

independent and dependent variables in your study.) So if you have a low *p*-value, that means the probability of finding those test results if the null hypothesis were true is very low. If your statistical test produces a high *p*-value, that means the probability of finding those test results if the null hypothesis were true is very high. If you look at the probability distribution in **Figure 3-9**, you can see that idea graphically. If your study examines the relationship between the number of hours spent in TED stockings and peripheral circulation, your null hypothesis would be: There is no relationship between the number of hours spent wearing TED stockings and peripheral circulation. After completing your analysis, you find that your test statistic has a *p*-value of 0.02. You can see that it is way out in the far end of the tail of the probability distribution. This is a pretty good sign that the probability of finding these test results, if your null hypothesis were true, is pretty small, and you may have enough evidence to support your alternative hypothesis that wearing TED stockings does

FIGURE 3-9   ***P*-values in a Probability Distribution.**

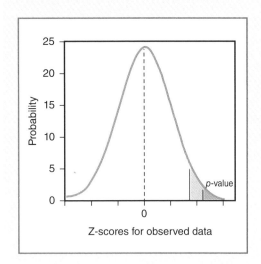

improve peripheral circulation. Determining if that probability level is statistically significant or not depends on a lot of other factors that we will talk about more later in the book. For now, just remember that when you hear *p*-value, it is the probability of finding the results you have if the null hypothesis were true. Most of the time, researchers want a low *p*-value because they really believe the alternative hypothesis is correct or they wouldn't have bothered with the study in the first place.

Let's spend a little more time looking at the difference between a frequency distribution and a probability distribution. The frequency distribution for the experiment of rolling a die 1,000 times is shown in **Figure 3-10** and compared against the probability distribution of rolling a die indefinitely. As you can see, the frequency distribution has notches and changes, depending on what a sample looks

like. The probability distribution is uniform and never changes. The relationship between relative frequency and probability closely resembles the relationship between a sample and a population. The difference boils down to a basic difference between the short run (100 tosses of the die) and the long run (1,000, 10,000, 100,000 tosses), and defining the long run is slightly subjective.

"That's great," you might say, "But I'm a nurse! I'm never going to need to roll dice and come up with associated probabilities unless I meet a poor statistician sitting at a bar all alone somewhere!" As it turns out, however, rolling a die is just a very straightforward example of

FIGURE 3-10 **Frequency versus Probability Distribution.**

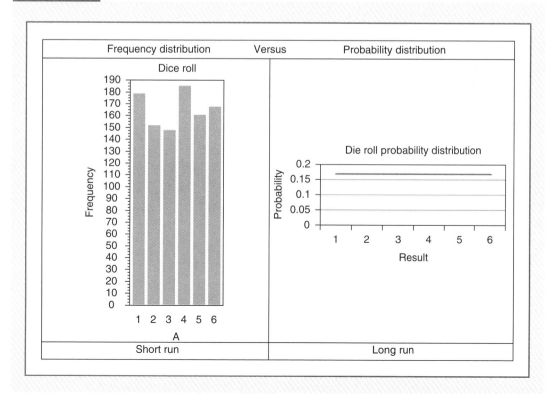

an experiment. Let's consider few questions and see how they might relate to your life and profession.

- What is the probability that I will die of cardiovascular disease?
- What is the probability that one of my patients will be discharged before I come back to the hospital to work my next shift?
- What is the probability that a new drug will kill a cancerous tumor in my patient's liver without killing my patient?

Answering these questions with any degree of accuracy requires a lot of study, a lot of repeated samples, and determining probability!

FIGURE 3-11   **Normal Distribution.**

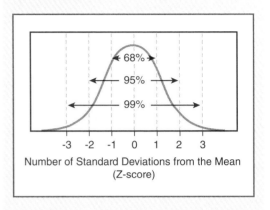

Number of Standard Deviations from the Mean (Z-score)

THE NORMAL DISTRIBUTION

Many variables of interest to us have a probability distribution that closely resembles a very famous distribution: the **normal distribution**, which is a probability distribution in which the mean, median, and mode are equal (see **Figure 3-11**). In fact, one of the most common assumptions in basic research is that the variables have probability distributions that can be estimated with the normal distribution. The normal distribution is also called the bell curve. And yes, this is how grades are "curved" when no one does well on a test. Many people believe that, given a well-constructed exam administered to a large enough sample, we should expect a grade distribution that can be estimated with the normal distribution.

Because the mean, median, and mode are the same in the normal distribution, you know

FROM THE STATISTICIAN *Brendan Heavey*

What Is a Normal Distribution?

For most researchers, the normal distribution is the most important distribution in all of statistics. Two very important facts about the normal distribution make it so important:

1. If you take the mean from lots and lots of samples of a population, the distribution of the sample means (the sampling distribution of the mean) becomes normal in the long run. **Sampling distributions** plot *actual* frequencies of a statistic versus the range of *possible* values that statistic can take.
2. As you add more and more random variables together, their overall distribution approaches the normal distribution.

Examine how the plot of the normal distribution in **Figure 3-12** looks as you adjust its mean. As the mean (μ) of the distribution increases in these graphs, the curve shifts to the right; as it decreases, the curve shifts to the left. This shift is why we call the mean a location parameter.

In **Figure 3-13**, see what happens when we change the variance. If we were to change only the variance (σ) in our formula, we would see a change in scale. As we decrease the variance, the graph gets taller and skinnier; as we increase it, the graph gets shorter and fatter. That is why variance is called a scale variable.

Here are some more important things we know about the normal distribution:

- Sixty-eight percent of the area under the curve falls within 1 standard deviation of the mean.
- Ninety-five percent of the area under the curve falls within 2 standard deviations of the mean.
- Increasing the mean makes the curve shift to the right.
- Decreasing the mean makes the curve shift to the left.
- Decreasing the variance makes the graph look taller and skinnier.
- Increasing the variance makes it look shorter and fatter.

An important thing we can do with any normal variable is transform its distribution into a *standard* normal distribution. This forces all the area under the curve to fall under the normal curve with a mean of 0 and a standard deviation of 1. We do this with the transformation formula shown in **Figure 3-14**. If Y is a normally distributed variable, this equation produces Z, which is a standard normal variable. Standard normal variables are great because we know a lot about their probabilities. For instance, 5% of the probability is found beyond $Z = 1.96$.

| FIGURE 3-12 | **Normal Distribution: Changing the Mean.** |

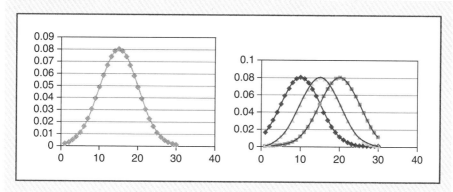

(continues)

FROM THE STATISTICIAN *Brendan Heavey*

FIGURE 3-13   **Normal Distribution: Changing the Variance.**

FIGURE 3-14   **Formula for Creating a Standard Normal Variable with Population Data.**

$$Z = \frac{Y - \mu}{\sigma} \sim N(0,1)$$

several things about a variable that is normally distributed (see Figure 3-11):

- Sixty-eight percent of its values fall within one standard deviation of the mean.
- Ninety-five percent of its values fall within two standard deviations of the mean.
- Ninety-nine percent of its values fall within three standard deviations of the mean.

SKEWED DISTRIBUTIONS

Of course, not all samples are normally distributed. For example, some samples are skewed; they have an asymmetrical distribution of the values of the variable around the mean so that one tail is longer than the other (see **Figure 3-15**). Skewing is usually due to a significant number

FIGURE 3-15   **Skewed Distributions.**

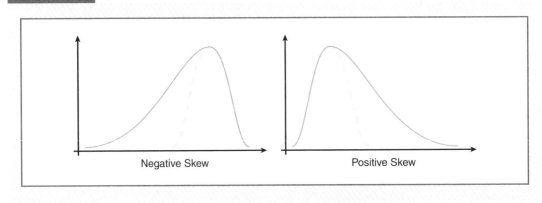

Negative Skew

Positive Skew

of outliers. When the outliers are on the right, the skew is positive; if most of the outliers are on the left, the skew is negative. In skewed distributions, the mean, median, and mode are not equal. Remember the test where you scored a 48 but only three people scored higher? That is an example of a positive skew produced by outliers.

Another interesting thing we can do when we have a normal distribution is to calculate a test statistic called a **Z-score**. A Z-score is a standardized measure that tells you how many standard deviations the observation is from the mean. If a value in a data set is above the mean or average, it will have a positive Z-score. If it is below the mean or average, it will have a negative Z-score. The larger the absolute value of the Z-score, the further the value is from the average or mean value in the data set. For example, a nurse educator gives a pretest to a group of newly diagnosed diabetics before teaching about insulin injection techniques. The test score is normally distributed, with an average score of 70% and a standard deviation of four points. The Z-score for a test value of 70% is 0, and a Z-score of 1.0 corresponds to a test score of 74%. A Z-score of 2.0 lies 2.0 standard deviations above the mean and, in this example, corresponds to a test score of 78%; in contrast, a Z-score of -0.5 lies 0.5 standard deviations below the mean, or, in this example, a test score of 68%. The formula for calculating Z-scores in a population is shown in Figure 3-14 and is just the observed value minus the mean, which is then divided by the standard deviation.

Z-scores can be helpful because we know the associated probability (such as 95%) of the values fall between two standard deviations or Z-scores of approximately -2 to $+2$. Z-scores are also standardized so we can use them to compare different values from different data sets. For example, an orthopedic rehabilitation

patient with a functional mobility test score of 12 and a corresponding Z-score value of 1, and a range of motion score of 17 with a corresponding Z-score of -0.5, means the patient is doing better than the population average in functional mobility but worse than the population average in range of motion. The absolute value of the test score does not tell us the relationship that this score may have to the usual or expected outcomes in the field, but a Z-score may give us that information.

SUMMARY

Congratulate yourself for making it through this chapter! Let's restate some main points from this very detailed chapter.

When you have nominal-level data, the only measure of central tendency you can use is the mode. The mode is the most frequently occurring measure in a distribution. A bimodal distribution has two values with the highest number of frequencies an equal number of times; this gives you two modes. A multimodal distribution has more than two modes.

The median can be used with ordinal, interval, or ratio data and is found by lining up the measured values, in order, from least to greatest and locating the value in the middle. For interval- or ratio-level data, you can also calculate a mean or average. The mean is the most commonly known measure of central tendency and is found by taking the sum of the values and dividing it by the total number of observations.

With regard to the dispersion of your data, two terms are important: (1) the range, or the difference between the maximum and minimum values in the distribution, and (2) the standard deviation, or the average distance of the values in a distribution from the center. We may choose to display the central tendency

FIGURE 3-16   **Box and Whiskers Plot with Turkey Fences.**

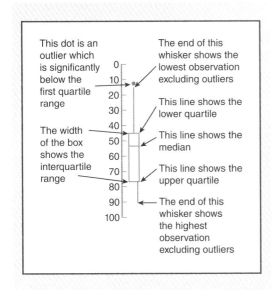

Modified from BBC. (2014). Maths: Statistics and probability. Retrieved from http://www.bbc.co.uk/schools/gcsebitesize/maths/statistics/representingdata3hirev6.shtml

and dispersion of our data graphically using a box and whiskers plot with Tukey fences. This may be helpful for identifying outliers and creating a visual representation of the data set.

Probability distributions also display graphically the range of observations made and the probability of each one occurring. This is very helpful because it helps us determine a p-value when statistical tests are utilized. A p-value is the probability of the observed results occurring if the null hypothesis is correct. A low p-value means there is a low probability of the results occurring if the null hypothesis is correct, and a high p value means there is a high probability of the results occurring if the null hypothesis is correct. This will come in very handy in another few chapters.

Everyone's favorite concept in statistics is the symmetrical normal distribution, often represented by the bell curve. If your data fits into this type of distribution, it simplifies your analysis immensely. It also lets you calculate Z-scores, which are standardized scores that can be useful in comparing different data sets.

Some samples are skewed; that is, they have an asymmetrical distribution of the values of the variable around the mean so that one tail is longer than the other. If you have this type of sample distribution, you need to make adjustments before applying some of the simpler analysis techniques.

If you understand these main concepts, you are on the right track and are ready to go on to the next chapter—or take a long nap. Personally, I would probably vote for the nap first anyhow!

CHAPTER 3 REVIEW QUESTIONS

Questions 1–5: Your results are 2, 14, 6, 8, 10, 4, 12, 8.

1. What is the mean?

2. What is the median?

3. What is the mode?

4. Calculate the standard deviation.

5. If the sample is normally distributed, 68% of the responses are within what range?

6. If a study reports that you have a normally distributed sample with a mean age of 17.3 years, what is the median?

Questions 7–12: A study polls 40 new mothers who attempt to nurse their infants from birth to 6 weeks. Twenty-seven mothers report nursing with minimal pain and frustration, 10 mothers report nursing with moderate pain and frustration, and 3 mothers report discontinuing nursing due to high levels of pain and frustration.

7. What is the mode for nursing pain and frustration?

8. What is the median for nursing pain and frustration?

9. What percentage of mothers continued to nurse for the full 6 weeks with minimal pain and frustration?

10. What percentage of mothers reported less than or equal to moderate pain and frustration?

11. What level of measurement is the nursing pain and frustration?

12. How could you increase the level of measurement?

Questions 13–18: You read a study involving a new screen for rheumatoid arthritis, and the report indicates that those with the disease had the antibody levels shown in **Table 3-3.**

13. Complete the cumulative frequency column.

14. How many subjects had their antibody levels reported?

15. What antibody level was the mode?

TABLE 3-3	**Frequency Table for Rheumatoid Arthritis Screen**	
Antibody Level	**Frequency**	**Cumulative Frequency**
20	3	—
30	5	—
43	3	—
48	7	—

16. What antibody level was the median?

17. What antibody level was the mean?

18. Is this sample normally distributed?

Questions 19–21: Final exam grades are normally distributed with a mean of 81. The standard deviation is 3.

19. What range includes 68% of the sample?

20. What range includes 95% of the sample?

21. What is the median grade?

Questions 22–26: A researcher is measuring how many times a minute a person coughs when exposed to cigarette smoke. The results from the study are normally distributed, and they include a mean of 4 and a standard deviation of 2.

22. What level of measurement is this?

23. What is an appropriate measure of central tendency?

24. Where do 68% of the sample responses fall?

25. If instead the results show a mean of 4 and a standard deviation of 1, but they remain normally distributed, what would this change do to the curve?

26. The follow-up cohort study reports a mean of 5 and a standard deviation of 1. What would this change do to the curve?

Questions 27–31: A sample of eight orthopedic patients on your unit includes two patients on intravenous anticoagulants, four patients on oral anticoagulants, and two patients on subcutaneous anticoagulants.

27. Based on this sample, calculate the probability that orthopedic patients are given IV anticoagulants.

28. Calculate the probability that orthopedic patients are given oral anticoagulants.

29. Calculate the probability that orthopedic patients are given subcutaneous anticoagulants.

30. Based on this sample, what is the probability that an orthopedic patient will be given some form of anticoagulant?

31. Hip replacement patients have the same probability of being on oral anticoagulants as the orthopedic patients in your previous study, and you have four in your daily assignment. Calculate the number of patients with hip replacements who you anticipate would need oral anticoagulants.

Questions 32–40: A researcher is comparing patients with high medication compliance versus those with low medication compliance in an outpatient psychiatric day program utilizing the Hamilton Anxiety Rating Scale (HAM-A), which has 14 items scored on a scale of 0–4. A higher score on the HAM-A indicates higher levels of anxiety. After collecting the data, she determines the scores obtained in both groups are normally distributed. In the low-compliance group, the mean score is 24 and the standard deviation is 2. In the high-compliance group, the mean score is 16 and the standard deviation is 1.5.

32. What level of measurement are the instrument items?

33. What is the median score in the low-compliance group?

34. A patient in the low-compliance group scores 26. Is this patient more or less anxious than average in this group?

35. Another patient in the low-compliance group has a score with a corresponding Z-score of -1.5. What was his actual HAM-A score? Was he more or less anxious than the average patient in this group?

36. The researcher knows that, with these results, 68% of her subjects in the low-compliance group scored in what range on the HAM-A?

37. A patient in the high-compliance group has a score with a corresponding Z-score of 2. What was her actual HAM-A score? Is she more or less anxious than the average patient in this group?

38. If the researcher graphs the frequency distributions for the scores in each of the two groups, which group will have a flatter bell curve? Why?

39. If instead of finding a normal distribution in the low-compliance group the researcher discovers there are three individuals with scores that are substantially higher than the rest of the group, what type of skew would these outliers cause?

40. If the distribution is skewed, what do you know about the mean, median, and mode?

41. Researchers run an analysis to determine if taking levothyroxine is associated with tachycardia. They report a p-value of 0.04. What general impression do you get from this result?

42. Researchers conduct a study to determine if there is a relationship between receiving the flu vaccine and developing the flu within 48 hours. They report a p-value of 0.78. What general impression do you get from this result?

ANSWERS TO ODD-NUMBERED CHAPTER 3 REVIEW QUESTIONS

1. 8

3. 8

5. Between 4 and 12

7. Minimal

9. 67.5%

11. Ordinal

13. 3, 8, 11, 18

15. Mode $= 48$

17. Mean $= 37.5$

19. 78–84

21. 81

23. Any

25. Make it taller and skinnier

27. $\frac{2}{8} = \frac{1}{4} = 25\%$

29. $\frac{2}{8} = \frac{1}{4} = 25\%$

31. 2

33. 24

35. 21, less anxious

37. 19, more anxious

39. Positive skew

41. There is a low probability that these results would occur if the null hypothesis is correct.

MEASURING DATA

IS YOUR STUDY GOOD, BAD, OR UGLY?

OBJECTIVES

By the end of the chapter students will be able to:

- Discuss factors that affect the feasibility of a study.

- Define validity, and explain why it is essential in research.

- Identify various methods for establishing validity, and give an example of each.

- Define reliability, and relate why it is important in research.

- Describe the main components of reliability.

- Detect when inter-rater reliability needs to be assessed, and develop a plan for doing so.

- Formulate a 2 × 2 table, and calculate the sensitivity and specificity of a screening test from a given data set.

- Distinguish between sensitivity and specificity, and identify when each is important.

- Calculate the positive and negative predictive values of a screening test.

- Calculate the prevalence of an illness, and describe how the positive and negative predictive values of the screening test are affected by the prevalence of the illness among the test population.

- Critique a screening test utilizing a given data set.

- Prepare an argument for why a particular screen should or should not be utilized based on current research.

KEY TERMS

Content validity
A determination that an instrument is designed to measure the concepts under study accurately.

Convergent validity
A determination that the test results obtained are similar to the results obtained with another previously validated test that measures the same thing.

Correlation coefficient
A test value used to determine how closely one measurement is related to a second measurement.

Cronbach's alpha
A measure of internal consistency reliability that ranges from 0 to 1. Higher values indicate greater internal consistency reliability.

Divergent validity
A determination that the measurement of the opposite variable of a previously validated measurement yields the opposite result.

Efficiency (EFF)
The probability of agreement between the screening test and the actual clinical diagnosis.

Equivalence
The measurement of how well multiple forms or multiple users of an instrument produce the same results.

Feasible
Possible from a practical standpoint.

Homogeneity
The extent to which items on a multi-item instrument are consistent with one another.

Internal consistency reliability
Homogeneity of the measurement instrument.

Inter-rater reliability
A comparison of the measurements obtained by two different data collectors to make sure they are similar.

Negative predictive value
The probability that a subject really doesn't have a disease when that subject tests negative for the disease.

Positive predictive value (PPV)
The probability that a subject actually has the disease when that subject tests positive for the disease.

Predictive validity
The measurement of how accurately an instrument suggests future outcomes or behaviors.

Prevalence
The amount of illness present in the population divided by the total population.

Reliability
The consistency or repeatability of the measurement.

Sensitivity
The probability of a positive test result for the disease (the probability of a true positive) if a patient has a disease.

Specificity
The probability that a well subject will have a negative screen (no disease) (the probability of a true negative).

Stability
The consistent or enduring quality of the measure.

Valid
Accurate.

Feasibility

Before selecting any type of research instrument, you should always assess how **feasible** or practical the tool is. For example, if you want to use computer-assisted interviewing techniques to survey adolescents about sexual behavior, but your grant is for $1,000 and each device costs $1,200, it is probably not a practical plan. A study that involves asking patients with dementia to complete a 24-hour recall of food consumption also lacks feasibility. In these cases, the researcher needs to take a moment for a quick reality check! Being a wise nurse, you know that you should always consider the feasibility or practical aspects of the study's measurement tool, such as the cost, time, training, and limitations of the study sample (physical, cultural, educational, psychosocial, etc.) before beginning the analysis of the validity and reliability of the instruments themselves.

Validity

After you determine that your instrument is feasible for use in your study, you can then proceed to assess the validity and reliability of your tool. The information you gather is helpful only if your measurement and collection methods are accurate, or **valid**. You can ensure that an instrument has validity in several ways:

- *Determine relevant variables by conducting a thorough literature search.* When you begin your research, conduct a literature search to determine what information, if any, is already available, for example, about the relationship between family visits and the length of recovery time needed after a hip replacement.

- *Include the variables in a measurement instrument.* In your literature search, identify some of the major variables to consider in your study, such as the support level of family members, the age of the patient, whether the patient lives alone, whether this was the patient's first surgery, and other factors.
- *Have your instrument reviewed by experts for feedback.* When you design the survey for your study, include the variables and then, for example, have your nurse manager, two nursing researchers, and your fellowship advisor (all experts) review your survey.

These steps are all part of ensuring **content validity**.

You can also show validity in your survey by comparing your results with those of a previously validated survey that measures the same thing. This type of comparison is called **convergent validity**. For example, if you find a correlation of 0.4 or higher, that finding strengthens the validity of both instruments, yours and the previous one (Grove, 2007). In turn, if your survey is later found to be able to predict the length of stay for those admitted in the future, that finding will strengthen the validity of your instrument, and your study would have **predictive validity** as well.

Some instruments are considered valid because they measure the opposite variable of a previously validated measurement and find the opposite result. For instance, suppose a group of people with elevated serum cholesterol levels also scored low on a survey you designed to measure intake of fruits and vegetables. This result is an example of **divergent validity** in your instrument. The group with high cholesterol also had a poor diet. If the negative correlation is greater than or equal to –0.4, the divergent validity of both measures is strengthened (Grove, 2007).

Another way to show validity with opposite results is if your instrument detects a difference in groups already known to have a difference. This is also referred to as construct validity testing using known groups. For example, you are testing a new instrument to examine labor outcomes in women who have already had a baby versus those experiencing their first labor. The instrument measures length of labor, which has already been shown to be shorter for women who have had a baby. You find that those who have had a baby have a length of labor that is on average 2 hours shorter than those who have not. This finding supports the validity of your new measurement tool because it detected a difference that was known to exist.

RELIABILITY

Reliability means that your measurement tool is consistent or repeatable. When you measure your variable of interest, do you get the same results every time? Reliability is different from accuracy or validity. Suppose, for example, that you are measuring the weight of the study participants, but your scale is not calibrated correctly: It is off by 20 pounds. You get the same measure every time the patient steps on the scale; that is, the measurement is repeatable and reliable. However, in this case, it is not accurate or valid. A measure can be reliable and not valid, but it can't be valid and not reliable. Think of it this way: For an instrument to be accurate (valid), it must be accurate and reliable.

Three main factors relate to reliability: stability, homogeneity, and equivalence. **Stability**

is the consistent or enduring quality of the measure. A stable measure:

- Should not change over time.
- Should have a high **correlation coefficient** when administered repeatedly. The correlation coefficient measures how closely one measurement is related to a second measurement. For example, if you measure the temperature of a healthy individual six times in an hour, the readings should be approximately the same and have a high correlation coefficient. (Of course, that patient may be really sick of having you around, but I am sure your excitement at discovering that you have a stable measure will make it all worthwhile!)

You need to evaluate the stability of your measurement instrument at the beginning of the study and throughout it. For example, if your thermometer breaks, the instrument that was once stable is no longer available. Your ongoing results are no longer reliable, and you need to have a protocol to figure out quickly how to reestablish stability.

The second quality of a reliable measure, **homogeneity**, is the extent to which items on a multi-item instrument are consistent with one another. For example, your survey may ask several questions designed to measure the level of family support. The questions may be repeated but worded differently to see whether the individuals completing the survey respond in the same way. One question may ask, "What level of family support do you feel on most days?" and the choices may be high, medium, and low. Later in the survey you may ask the individual to indicate on a scale of 1 to 10 the degree of family support felt on an average day. If the instrument has homogeneity, those who answered that they had, say, a medium level of family support on most days should also be somewhere around the middle of the 1–10 scale. If so, then your instrument is said to have **internal consistency reliability**.

Internal consistency reliability is useful for instruments that measure a single concept, such as family support, and is frequently assessed using **Cronbach's alpha**. Cronbach's alpha ranges from 0 (no reliability in the instrument scale) to 1 (perfect reliability in the instrument scale), so a higher value indicates better internal consistency reliability. You may hear more about this test in future statistics or research classes, but right now you just need to know that it can be used to establish homogeneity or internal consistency reliability (Nieswiadomy, 2008).

The third factor relating to reliability is **equivalence**. Equivalence is how well multiple forms of an instrument or multiple users of an instrument produce/obtain the same results. Measurement variation is a reflection of more than the reliability of the tool itself; it may also reflect the variability of different forms of the tool or variability due to different researchers administering the same tool. For example, if you want to observe the color of scrubs worn by 60 nurses at lunchtime on a particular day, you might need help in gathering that much data in such a short period of time. You might ask two research assistants to observe the nurses. When you have more than one individual collecting data, you should determine the **inter-rater reliability**. One way to do this is to have all three individuals who are collecting data observe the first five nurses together and then classify the data individually. For example:

- You say the first five nurses are wearing blue, green, green, orange, and pink scrubs.

- The second research assistant reports that the first five nurses are wearing teal, lime, lime, tangerine, and rose scrubs.
- The third reports that the first five nurses are wearing blue, green, green, orange, and pink scrubs.

In this example, the inter-rater reliability between you and the third data collector is 100%, whereas it is 0% between you and the second collector. You have clearly identified a problem with the instrument's inter-rater reliability.

One way to increase reliability is to create color categories for data collection, for example, blue, green, orange, yellow, and other. In this case:

- You report the first five nurses are wearing blue, green, green, orange, and other.
- The second data collector reports the nurses are wearing blue, green, green, other, and other.
- The third data collector matches your selections again.

Clearly you have improved the inter-rater reliability, but some variability is left due to the collectors' differences in interpretation of colors. With this information, you may decide that the help of the second data collector isn't worth the loss in inter-rater reliability. You might run the study with only two data collectors, or you may decide to sit down, define specific colors with the second data collector, and then reexamine the inter-rater reliability. In all such cases, you must consider this concern whenever the study requires more than one data collector.

The readability of an instrument can also affect both the validity and the reliability of the tool. If your study participants cannot understand the words in your survey tool, there is a very good chance they will not complete it accurately or consistently, which would ruin all your hard work. A good researcher assesses the readability of his or her instrument before or during the pilot stage of a study.

One last point to remember is that the validity and reliability of an instrument are not inherent attributes of the instrument but are characteristics of the use of the instrument with a particular group of respondents at a particular time. For example, an instrument that has been shown to be valid and reliable when used with an urban elderly population may not be valid and reliable when used with a rural adolescent population. For this reason, the validity and reliability of an instrument should be reassessed whenever that instrument is used in a new situation.

SCREENING TESTS

Different but related terms are utilized when a screening test is selected. The accuracy of a screening test is determined by its ability to identify subjects who have the disease and subjects who do not. However, accuracy does not mean that all subjects who have a positive screen have the disease and that all subjects who have a negative screen do not.

The four possible outcomes from any screening test are best illustrated in a standard 2 × 2 table, also called a contingency table (see **Figure 4-1**).

FIGURE 4-1   **A 2 × 2 Table.**

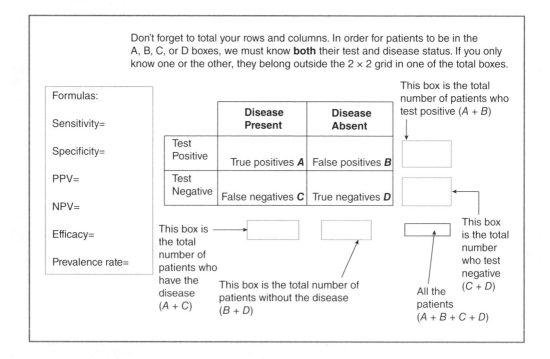

- If a subject actually has the disease and the screen is positive, the result is a true positive and belongs in the first box (*A*).
- If the subject does not have the disease and the screen is positive, it is a false positive and belongs in the second box (*B*).
- If the subject has the disease and tests negative, it is a false negative and belongs in the third box (*C*).
- If the subject does not have the disease and the screen is negative, it is a true negative and belongs in the fourth box (*D*).

Don't forget to total your rows and columns. In order for patients to be in the *A*, *B*, *C*, or *D* boxes, we must know *both* their test and disease status. If you know only one or the other for a patient, that patient belongs outside the 2 × 2 grid in one of the total boxes.

SENSITIVITY

When evaluating a screening test, one of the things nurses like to know is the probability that a patient will test positive for the disease, if the patient has the disease. This is known as the **sensitivity** of the test and can be calculated by the equation in **Figure 4-2**. This equation should make sense. Take the number of subjects who are sick and test positive, and divide this number by the total number of subjects who are ill. It is

a matter of percentages: the number of patients who are really sick and who test positive divided by the total number of people who really are sick. If a screen is sensitive, it is very good at identifying people who are actually sick, and it has a low percentage of false negatives. Sensitivity is particularly important when a disease is fatal or contagious or when early treatment helps.

SPECIFICITY

Another piece of information that helps evaluate a screening tool is the **specificity**, or the probability that a well subject will have a negative screen (no disease). Using the same 2 × 2 table, specificity can be calculated with the equation in **Figure 4-3**. Similar to the previous equation, this equation takes the number of people who are not ill and who have a negative screening test and divides this number by the total number of people who are not ill. When a screen is highly specific, it is very good at identifying subjects who are not ill, and it has a low percentage of false positives. Specificity is particularly important if you have transient subjects and it would be difficult to find them again in the future.

Sensitivity and specificity tend to work in a converse balance with each other, and sometimes a loss in one is traded for an improvement in another. For example, suppose you are a nurse

FIGURE 4-2 | **Formula to Calculate the Sensitivity of a Screen.**

$$\text{Sensitivity} = \frac{A\,(\text{True positives})}{A + C\,(\text{All who have the disease})}$$

FIGURE 4-3 | **Formula to Calculate the Specificity of a Screen.**

$$\text{Sensitivity} = \frac{\text{True negatives}\,(D)}{\text{All those who do not have the disease}\,(B + D)}$$

working on an infectious disease outbreak in a mobile military unit overseas. Your ability to find these patients again is very limited, so you want to be as certain as possible that those you screen negative and who leave the mobile facility are not really carrying the disease for which you are screening. Thus, you select a highly specific test that is very good at identifying those who do not have the disease for which you are screening. When a highly specific test is negative, you know the chances are very good that the person is actually healthy and can leave the facility without a concern that she or he could spread the disease for which you are screening. You can then hold or contain those who do test positive for further testing and evaluation.

FROM THE STATISTICIAN *Brendan Heavey*

Sensitivity and Specificity

Let's review some concepts in this chapter in the context of testing a large group of individuals for tuberculosis. For instance, when you entered nursing school, you were probably subjected to tests to determine whether you were ever infected with tuberculosis. The first step in the testing process is a purified protein derivative (PPD), which shows whether a person has antibodies to the bacterium that causes tuberculosis. A person with a positive response to this test may be asked to undergo any number of tests, including:

- Serological testing
- Chest x-ray
- Biopsy
- Urine culture
- Cerebrospinal fluid sample
- Computed tomography (CT) scan
- Magnetic resonance imaging (MRI) scan

Each of these tests has a number of different characteristics. They can all be used in the diagnosis of tuberculosis, but which test is best?

This question turns out to be very challenging, and the answer depends on the definition of "best." In addition, each person's definition of best can be different and can change depending on that individual's perception of reality. For instance, each test costs a different amount to administer, so is the cheapest test the best? (If you thought you had tuberculosis, cost would probably not be your criterion for best.) Each test also ranges in its degree of invasiveness. Would you want to be subjected to a cerebrospinal fluid sample (which is very painful) if you didn't think you had the disease and just wanted to get into nursing school?

Each of these tests has a different sensitivity and specificity. A very important trait of each test that you should be interested in knowing is how often a person with tuberculosis is actually diagnosed correctly. A second trait of interest

FROM THE STATISTICIAN *Brendan Heavey*

is how often a person without tuberculosis is correctly diagnosed. In general, a high-sensitivity/lower-specificity test is administered first to determine a large set of people who *may* have the disease. Sensitive tests are very good at identifying those who have a disease. Then additional costs and tests are incurred to increase specificity, or eliminate people who are actually healthy (and were false positives) before diagnosis and treatment begin.

This approach is like using a microscope. The first step is to use a low-resolution lens to find the area of a slide that you are interested in. Then you increase the resolution to look more closely at the object of interest. A test with high sensitivity/low specificity is like a low-resolution lens to identify those who may have the disease. As you increase specificity, you narrow down the population of interest and eliminate those who were falsely testing positive. An example of this practice is included in Doering et al. (2007).

POSITIVE PREDICTIVE VALUE OF A SCREEN

Another important concept to understand about any screening test is **positive predictive value (PPV)**. PPV tells you what the probability is that a subject actually has the disease given a positive test result—that is, the probability of a true positive. Look back at the 2 × 2 table in Figure 4-1. You can calculate the PPV with the equation in **Figure 4-4**.

Many students find this concept confusing because it depends not just on the sensitivity and specificity of the test but also on the **prevalence** of the illness in the population being screened. Prevalence is the amount of illness (the number of cases) present in the population divided by the total population. If you look back at the 2 × 2 table, you can determine the prevalence quite easily. It is just the number of people who have the disease divided by the total population (see **Figure 4-5**).

If you administer a screening test with an established sensitivity and specificity in a population with a low prevalence of the disease, your screening test will have a low positive

FIGURE 4-4 **Formula to Calculate the Positive Predictive Value of a Screen.**

$$PPV = \frac{\text{True positives } (A)}{\text{Total number who tested positive } (A+B)}$$

FIGURE 4-5 **Formula to Calculate Prevalence from a 2 × 2 Table.**

$$\text{Prevalence} = \frac{\text{All with the disease } (A+C)}{\text{Entire sample } (A+B+C+D)}$$

FIGURE 4-6   **Application of Screen in a Sample with a 5% Prevalence Rate.**

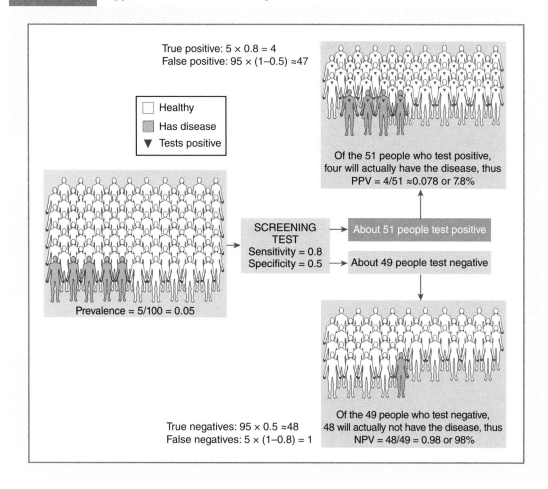

True positive: 5 × 0.8 = 4
False positive: 95 × (1–0.5) ≈47

Healthy
Has disease
▼ Tests positive

Of the 51 people who test positive,
four will actually have the disease, thus
PPV = 4/51 ≈0.078 or 7.8%

Prevalence = 5/100 = 0.05

SCREENING
TEST
Sensitivity = 0.8
Specificity = 0.5

About 51 people test positive

About 49 people test negative

Of the 49 people who test negative,
48 will actually not have the disease, thus
NPV = 48/49 = 0.98 or 98%

True negatives: 95 × 0.5 ≈48
False negatives: 5 × (1–0.8) = 1

Based on Genomes Unzipped. (2010). *How well can a screening test predict disease risk?* Retrieved from http://genomesunzipped
.org/2010/08/predictive-capacity-of-screening-tests.php

predictive value. Let's look at an example. If you apply a screen with a sensitivity of 80% and a specificity of 50% to a population with a prevalence rate of 5%, your PPV will be only 7.8%. (See **Figure 4-6**.)

However, if you administer the same test with the same sensitivity and specificity in a population where 25% of the population has the condition, your screening will have a heightened positive predictive value of 35.1%. Even without looking at the 2 × 2 table, this phenomenon makes sense. If you are looking for a disease that is very rare, a positive test result in that population is more likely to be a

| FIGURE 4-7 | **Application of Screen in a Sample with a 25% Prevalence Rate.** |

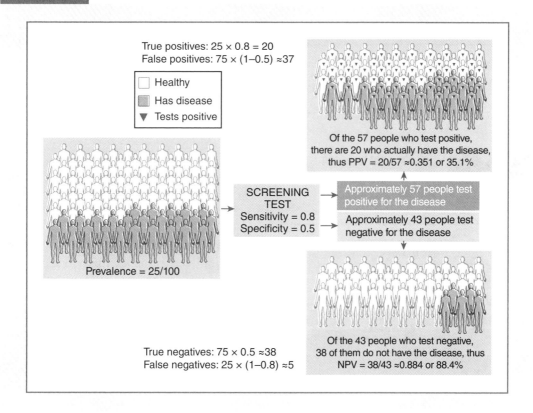

True positives: 25 × 0.8 = 20
False positives: 75 × (1–0.5) ≈37

☐ Healthy
▨ Has disease
▼ Tests positive

Of the 57 people who test positive,
there are 20 who actually have the disease,
thus PPV = 20/57 ≈0.351 or 35.1%

SCREENING
TEST
Sensitivity = 0.8
Specificity = 0.5

Approximately 57 people test
positive for the disease

Approximately 43 people test
negative for the disease

Prevalence = 25/100

Of the 43 people who test negative,
38 of them do not have the disease, thus
NPV = 38/43 ≈0.884 or 88.4%

True negatives: 75 × 0.5 ≈38
False negatives: 25 × (1–0.8) ≈5

Based on Genomes Unzipped. (2010). How well can a screening test predict disease risk? Retrieved from http://genomesunzipped
.org/2010/08/predictive-capacity-of-screening-tests.php

false positive than in a population where 25% of the population actually has the disease. When prevalence increases, PPV increases, and vice versa (**Figure 4-7**). The two measures travel together in the same direction.

NEGATIVE PREDICTIVE VALUE

A related concept is the **negative predictive value (NPV)** of a test: If your subject screens negatively, NPV tells you the probability that the patient really does not have the disease.

Like PPV, this measure depends on sensitivity, specificity, and the prevalence of the illness in the population where you are administering the test. Using the 2 × 2 table again, you can determine the NPV using the equation in **Figure 4-8**. With our previous example, you will see that when the prevalence of the disease is 5%, the NPV is 98%, (see Figure 4-6) but when the prevalence is higher, and 25% of the sample has the condition, the NPV decreases to 88.4% (see Figure 4-7). Again, this makes sense; when very few people have the condition,

FIGURE 4-8   **Formula to Calculate Negative Predictive Value (NPV) from a 2 × 2 Table.**

$$NPV = \frac{\text{True negatives }(D)}{\text{All the subjects who tested negative }(C+D)}$$

FIGURE 4-10   **Formula for Calculating Efficiency (EFF).**

$$EFF = \frac{\text{All accurate test results }(A+D)}{\text{Entire sample }(A+B+C+D)}$$

FIGURE 4-9   **Relationship between Prevalence and Predictive Values.**

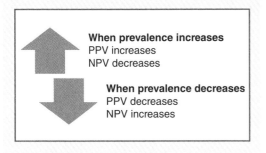

When prevalence increases
PPV increases
NPV decreases

When prevalence decreases
PPV decreases
NPV increases

a negative screen is more likely to be accurate. When quite a few people have the condition, a negative screen is less likely to be accurate. Prevalence and NPV are measures that travel in opposite directions (see **Figure 4-9**).

EFFICIENCY

One last concept is particularly useful in a clinical setting. **Efficiency (EFF)** is a measure of the agreement between the screening test and the actual clinical diagnosis. To determine efficiency, add all the true positives and all the true negatives, and determine what proportion of your sample that is. (This proportion is the group that the test correctly identified, and therefore the diagnosis is made correctly. That is always a good thing in nursing!) Efficiency can be calculated by using the formula in **Figure 4-10**.

SUMMARY

You have completed the chapter and are doing a great job! Let's recap the main ideas.

Validity is the accuracy of your measurement. To assess content validity, determine the relevant variables from a thorough literature search, include them in your measurement instrument, and have your instrument reviewed by experts for feedback. For convergent validity, compare your results with those of another previously validated survey that measured the same thing. Divergent validity is the opposite: It measures the opposite variable of a previously validated measurement and finds the opposite result.

Reliability tells you whether your measurement tool is consistent or repeatable. Stability is one of the main factors that contribute to reliability and is the consistent or enduring quality of the measure. Another component or type of reliability is homogeneity or the extent to which items on a multi-item instrument are consistent with one other. Also, equivalence reliability tells you whether multiple forms or multiple users of an instrument produce the same results.

Nurses like to know the sensitivity and specificity of screening tests. Sensitivity is the probability of getting a true positive, and specificity is the probability of getting a true negative. The prevalence of the illness in a population affects the positive and negative predictive values of a screening test.

Again, great work for completing this difficult chapter. If you are somewhat confused by these new concepts, continue to practice, practice, practice! Believe it or not, you will look back on these concepts at the end of the semester, and they will make sense.

CHAPTER 4 REVIEW QUESTIONS

1. Your test is very good at correctly identifying when a person actually has a disease. Your test a measure of which of the following?
   a. sensitivity
   b. specificity
   c. collinearity
   d. effect size

2. If a person has a disease and tests positive for it, the result is an example of which of the following?
   a. a true negative
   b. a false positive
   c. a false negative
   d. a true positive

Questions 3–4: You are studying a new screening test. Of the 100 people who do not have a disease, 80 test negative for it with your new screen. Of the 100 people who do have the disease, 90 test positive with your screen.

3. The sensitivity of your screen is _____.

4. Your new screen's specificity is _____.

5. You have a new tool that examines outcomes in pregnancy. A previously validated tool reports that cesarean section rates in your area are 30%. The correlation between the old tool and your tool is 0.7. This result indicates which of the following?
   a. convergent validity
   b. content validity
   c. divergent validity
   d. validity from contrasting groups

Questions 6–13: You are developing a new screening test and construct the test results shown in **Table 4-1**.

TABLE 4-1	**A 2 × 2 Table**		
	Disease Present	**Disease Not Present**	**Totals**
Test Positive	44	3	47
Test Negative	6	97	103
Totals	50	100	150

6. How many true positives do you have?

7. Without using statistics jargon, explain what each box represents.

8. What is the sensitivity of your new test?

9. What is the specificity of your new test?

10. Give an example of a clinical situation in which this might be a good test to use.

11. What is the positive predictive value of your screening test?

12. What is the prevalence of the disease you are testing for?

13. If this disease were fatal, would you be concerned about this prevalence rate?

Research Application

Questions 14–17: A small study was done to compare the results from three different chlamydia screening tests. The results obtained are shown in **Table 4-2**.

| TABLE 4-2 | A 2 × 2 Table for Chlamydia Screen |

	Sensitivity	Specificity	PPV	NPV
Screen *A*	57	96	66	94
Screen *B*	85	82	37	98
Screen *C*	57	94	57	94

14. Which screen has the lowest specificity? Why might it still be a good screen to use?

15. Which screen has the highest positive predictive value? If you administered this screen in a population with a high prevalence, what would you expect to happen to the positive predictive value?

16. If you know that early treatment helps prevent infertility and that chlamydia is very contagious, would sensitivity or specificity be more important to you? With that in mind, which of these tests would you prefer to utilize?

17. If all the tests are administered in the same manner and cost the same, which one would you recommend that your clinic use? Justify your answer.

Questions 18–23: You are using a screening test in your clinic to detect abnormal cervical cells related to the presence of human papilloma virus (HPV). Your results are shown in **Table 4-3**.

TABLE 4-3	**Screen Test Results**		
	Abnormal Cells Present	**Abnormal Cells Not Present**	**Totals**
Test Positive	360	20	380
Test Negative	40	80	120
Totals	400	100	500

18. What is the prevalence of abnormal cells in your clinic? What does this mean in nonstatistical language, or plain English?

19. What is the sensitivity of the screen? What does this mean in nonstatistical language, or plain English?

20. What is the specificity of the screen? What does this mean in nonstatistical language, or plain English?

21. What is the positive predictive value (PPV) of the screen? What does this mean in nonstatistical language, or plain English?

22. What is the negative predictive value (NPV) of the screen? What does this mean in nonstatistical language, or plain English?

23. What is the efficiency of the screen? What does this mean in nonstatistical language, or plain English?

Questions 24–31: A new vaccine is developed that provides immunity to the virus causing abnormal cervical cells, and you reexamine data 2 years after the vaccine is implemented at your clinic. See the results in **Table 4-4**.

TABLE 4-4	**Screening Test Results after Vaccine Implementation**		
	Abnormal Cells Present	**Abnormal Cells Not Present**	**Totals**
Test Positive	180	60	240
Test Negative	20	240	260
Totals	200	300	500

24. What is the prevalence of abnormal cervical cells after the vaccine is utilized? How did the vaccine affect the prevalence?

25. What is the sensitivity of the screen? Does a change in prevalence affect the sensitivity?

26. What is the specificity of the screen? Does a change in prevalence affect the specificity?

27. What is the PPV of the screen? Does a change in prevalence affect the PPV? How?

28. What is the NPV of the screen? Does a change in prevalence affect the NPV? How?

29. What happens to the number of false positives when the prevalence rates go down?

30. What happens to the efficiency of the screen when the prevalence rates go down?

31. Why might you consider lengthening the time between screens or developing a more specific screen with the new prevalence rate?

_____

_____

32. Melanomas are the deadliest form of skin cancer, affecting more than 53,000 Americans each year and killing more than 7,000 annually. Your state currently has 167 cases of melanoma reported, and there are 1,420,000 people in the state. What is the prevalence rate in your state?

_____

_____

Questions 33–39: A clinical study is established to determine if the results of a screening stress test can be used as a predictor of the presence of heart disease. The study enrolls 100 participants who undergo a screening stress test and then have their disease state confirmed by an angiogram (gold standard). Twenty participants screened positive with their stress tests and had confirmed heart disease on their angiogram. One participant who screened positive on his stress test had a normal angiogram and did not have heart disease. Seventy-seven participants screened negative on their stress tests and had normal angiograms without heart disease.

33. Develop an appropriate 2 $\times$ 2 table illustrating this information.

_____

_____

34. What is the sensitivity of the screening stress test? What does this mean in nonstatistical language, or plain English?

_____

_____

35. What is the specificity of the screening stress test? What does this mean in nonstatistical language, or plain English?

_____

_____

36. What is the PPV of the screening stress test? What does this mean in nonstatistical language, or plain English?

_____

_____

37. What is the NPV of the screening stress test? What does this mean in nonstatistical language, or plain English?

_____

_____

38. What is the disease prevalence in this sample?

_____

_____

39. What is the efficacy of this screen?

_____

_____

40. You have developed a new buccal swab test for hepatitis C and enroll 1,388 subjects to test the screen. There are 941 people who do not have hepatitis C and test negative with your screen. There are 388 people who test positive with your screen. There are 435 subjects with confirmed cases of hepatitis C, and 59 test negative. Complete the appropriate 2 × 2 table and use it to answer the following questions.

Table for Screening Test for Hepatitis

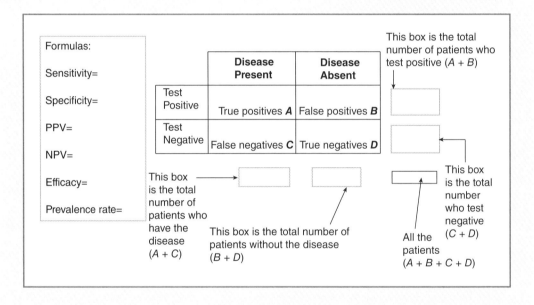

41. You are studying a new screening instrument and determine the following after screening 135 people. Of the 60 individuals who are known to have the disease, 58 screen positive. One person without the disease screens positive. Seventy-four people without the disease screen negative. Which of the following statements is true?
    a. The disease has a negatively correlated attack rate of 44%.
    b. Each additional exposure is likely to be associated with a sevenfold increase in your outcome variable.
    c. The efficiency of the screen is approximately 88%.
    d. If a person screens positive, there is a 97% chance that he or she actually has the disease.

42. You are studying a new screening instrument and determine the following after screening 135 people. Of the 60 individuals who are known to have the disease, 58 screen positive. One person without the disease screens positive. Seventy-four people without the disease screen negative. Which of the following statements is true?
    a. The disease has a negatively correlated attack rate of 44%.
    b. Each additional exposure is likely to be associated with a tenfold increase in your outcome variable.
    c. If the person screens negative, there is a 99% chance that he or she does not have the disease.
    d. If a person screens positive, there is a 77% chance that he or she actually has the disease.

43. You are studying a new screening instrument and determine the following after screening 135 people. Of the 60 individuals who are known to have the disease, 58 screen positive. One person without the disease screens positive. Seventy-four people without the disease screen negative. Which of the following statements is true?
    a. The specificity of the screen is higher than the sensitivity of the screen.
    b. Each additional exposure is likely to be associated with a 10-fold increase in your outcome variable.
    c. If the person screens negative, there is a 79% chance that he or she does not have the disease.
    d. If a person screens positive, there is a 77% chance that he or she actually has the disease.

44. You are studying a new screening instrument and determine the following after screening 135 people. Of the 60 individuals who are known to have the disease, 58 screen positive. One person without the disease screens positive. Seventy-four people without the disease screen negative. What is the efficiency of the screening test?
    a. 98%
    b. 96%
    c. 99%
    d. 44%

ANSWERS TO ODD-NUMBERED CHAPTER 4 REVIEW QUESTIONS

1. a

3. 90%

5. a

7. 44 true positives, 3 false positives, 47 all positive tests, 6 false negatives, 97 true negatives, 103 all negative tests, 50 total with disease, 100 healthy total, 150 total population

9. 97 ÷ 100, 97%

11. 44 ÷ 47, 93.6%

13. Yes! A third of the population has the disease. That is a substantial disease burden.

15. A, high prevalence increases PPV; therefore, the PPV would increase.

17. Answers will vary but should not include screen C, which has lower specificity and PPV than screen A and the same sensitivity and NPV.

19. 360 ÷ 400, 90% (If the patient has abnormal cervical cells, there is a 90% probability that the screen will be positive and detect the abnormal cells.)

21. 360 ÷ 380, 94.7% (Of all the patients who screen positive, 94.7% are patients who really have abnormal cervical cells.)

23. 440 ÷ 500, 88% (Eighty-eight percent of the time, the screen correctly identifies the patient's disease state.)

25. 180 ÷ 200, 90% (stays the same)

27. 180 ÷ 240, 75% (PPV decreases when prevalence goes down! You are more likely to have false positives in areas with lower prevalence.)

29. False positives increase.

31. Answers will vary but should include: False positives create a financial burden because unnecessary services are provided. Also, there may be negative health impacts from the stress, anxiety, loss of work time, and any other unnecessary screens or procedures that result from the false positive screen.

33.

	Disease Is Present	**No Disease**	**Total**
Screen test positive	20	1	21
Screen test negative	2	77	79
Total	22	78	100

35. 77/78, 98.7%. When a subject does not have the disease, there is a 98.7% chance the screening test will say that he or she is disease-free.

37. 77/79, 97.5%. When a subject has a negative screening stress test, there is a 97.5% chance he or she does not have the disease.

39. 97/100, 97%

41. d

43. a

CHAPTER 5

SAMPLING METHODS

DOES THE SAMPLE REPRESENT THE POPULATION?

OBJECTIVES

By the end of this chapter students will be able to:

- Compare and contrast probability and nonprobability sampling, and describe at least one example of each.

- Identify similarities and differences among simple random sampling, systematic sampling, stratified sampling, and cluster sampling.

- Identify sampling error, contrast it with sampling bias, and identify the effect of each.

- Explain why the central limit theorem is useful in statistics.

- Identify situations in which nonprobability sampling is utilized and what limits are created by doing so.

- Given a research proposal, compose inclusion and exclusion criteria.

- Evaluate sampling techniques' strengths and weaknesses in a current research article.

KEY TERMS

Cluster sampling
Probability sampling using a group or unit rather than an individual.

Convenience sampling
A form of nonprobability sampling that consists of collecting data from the group that is available.

Exclusion criteria
The list of characteristics that would eliminate a subject from being eligible to participate in a study.

Inclusion criteria
The list of characteristics a subject must have to be eligible to participate in a study.

Nonprobability sampling
Methods in which subjects do not have the same chance of being selected for participation (not randomized).

Probability sampling
Techniques in which the probability of selecting each subject is known (randomized).

Quota sampling
A form of nonprobability sampling in which you select the proportions of the sample for different subgroups, much the same as in stratified sampling but without random selection.

Sampling bias
A systematic error made in the sample selection that results in a nonrandom sample.

Sampling distribution
All the possible values of a statistic from all the possible samples of a given population.

Sampling error
Differences between the sample and the population that occur due to randomization or chance.

Sampling method
The processes employed to select the subjects for a sample from the population being studied.

Simple random sampling
Probability sampling in which every subject in a population has the same chance of being selected.

Stratified sampling
Probability sampling that divides the population into subsamples according to a characteristic of interest and then randomly selects the sample from these subgroups.

Systematic sampling
Probability sampling involving the selection of subjects according to a standardized rule.

SAMPLING METHODS

Let's look at the concepts of populations and samples. When you begin your nursing research, you develop a hypothesis that reflects what you think is occurring in a particular population. For example, your hypothesis might be: Men with heart disease die earlier than men without heart disease. Your population is the whole group that is of interest to you, in this case, all adult men. Although you are an amazing nurse researcher, measuring the life spans of all men is impossible. Instead, you decide to collect a representative sample of these men to study. To be representative of the population, the sample must reflect its important characteristics. For example, if 50% of adult men are over 60 years old, 50% of your sample should also be men over 60 years old. Your sample, then, is a group of subjects selected from the population for the purpose of conducting your research. Because your sample is representative, you can complete your study and then develop inferences about the impact of heart disease on the entire population of men from your sample of men.

The **sampling method** you will use consists of the processes of selecting the subjects for your sample from the population under study. Of the many kinds of sampling methods, the one you select depends a great deal on your population of interest and on the options available to you at the time. There are two main kinds of sampling methods: probability sampling and nonprobability sampling. Both methods are of value to researchers. Determining the best sampling method to utilize in a study involves determining the feasibility of the method, the best way to answer the research question, and the resources that are available to do so.

PROBABILITY SAMPLING

Probability sampling consists of techniques in which the probability of selecting each subject is known. Because this type of sampling requires the researcher to identify every member of the population, it is frequently not feasible with large populations. It can be accomplished in a number of ways, including simple random sampling, systematic sampling, stratified sampling, and cluster sampling. All of these methods of probability sampling involve randomization of some sort. That is a key idea in probability sampling.

SIMPLE RANDOM SAMPLING

With **simple random sampling**, every subject in a population has the same chance of being selected. Suppose you wish to determine the mean age of the nurses at your hospital. You could use a list of all hospital nurses ($n = 100$) and then *randomly* select 50 subjects from the list for your sample. As long as the selection is from all 100 nurses each time, the probability of selecting each individual is exactly the same (1/100). Although simple random sampling is ideal, it doesn't work without a limited and very well-defined population of interest.

SYSTEMATIC SAMPLING

A similar approach, **systematic sampling**, involves *randomly* selecting your subjects according to a standardized rule. One way of doing this is to number the whole population again, pick a random starting point, and then select every nth person. For example, you might take the same list of 100 nurses from your hospital and randomly start with the 17th nurse on the list and then select every 9th one. When using this approach, you have to make sure the population list is not developed with any ranking order. For example, if your list is arranged by clinical track levels for each unit, the ninth person may fall into about the same track level consistently, and that may be an achievement related to age. Your sample would then not be representative of the population of nurses working at your hospital.

STRATIFIED SAMPLING

Stratified sampling divides the population into subsamples according to a characteristic of interest and then *randomly* selects the sample from these subgroups. The purpose is to ensure representativeness of the characteristic. An example should make that clearer. You are still trying to determine the average age of the nurses in your hospital, but you know that how long the nurses have practiced is related to their age, and you want to make sure that your sample reflects this population characteristic. You are aware that 20% of the nurses have been practicing for 1 year or less, and the rest have more than 1 year of experience. You decide to use stratified random sampling to make sure your sample is representative of the population in terms of working experience. So you identify the nurses at the hospital with 1 year or less experience and *randomly* select 20% of your sample from this group and then *randomly* select 80% of your sample from the group of nurses who have more than 1 year of experience.

CLUSTER SAMPLING

Cluster sampling randomly selects a group or unit rather than an individual. It is used when it is difficult to find a list of the entire population. If, for example, you wanted to know the mean income of adults living in New York State, you may choose to select randomly four ZIP code areas, survey everyone over age 18 in each of those regions, and take a weighted-average score. Or if you wanted

to know the mean age of nurses employed in hospitals in New York, you may decide to select randomly a sample of hospitals in New York (each hospital is a cluster or group) and then find out the age of all the nurses at those hospitals.

If that approach is too difficult, you can do two-staged cluster sampling. You would randomly select the four hospitals in New York, and then, rather than taking the age of each nurse at the cluster hospitals, you would again take a random sample of a group of nurses at each hospital. In effect, you randomly selected your clusters and then randomly selected your final sample from each of these clusters. Although less expensive than other methods, cluster sampling has its drawbacks in terms of statistics (greater variance), but it is sometimes a necessary approach (Pagano & Gauvreau, 1993).

SAMPLING ERROR VERSUS SAMPLING BIAS

No matter which random sampling technique you choose for your study, there will always be some **sampling error**, that is, some differences between the sample and the population that occur due to chance. Anytime you are examining a random sample and not the whole population, you will encounter some differences that are not under your control and that occur only because of randomization or chance. That is why inferences made from sample data about a population are always made as probability statements, not absolutes.

Sampling error is not the same as **sampling bias**, which is a systematic error made in the sample selection that results in a nonrandom sample. In the previous example, you decided to take a systematic sample from a list of nurses at your hospital to determine the mean number of years they worked at your hospital. Unfortunately, you did not realize that the list was arranged by clinical track levels for each unit. You chose to start at the beginning and sample every ninth person. Unfortunately, the ninth person fell in about the same track level consistently, and track levels are related to the number of years worked at the hospital. Your results had a significant amount of sampling bias and were not representative of the population of interest; therefore, your results should not be generalized to the original population.

SAMPLING DISTRIBUTIONS

Talking about the benefits of random sampling can get a little statistical, but bear with me. Suppose you collect a random sample of nurses from a population of nurses, calculate the mean age, and keep doing this with other random samples of nurses from the same population. Eventually you will develop a distribution of the mean age. This is your **sampling distribution**, which consists of all the possible values of a statistic from all the possible samples of a given population (Corty, 2007). See **Table 5-1** and **Figure 5-1**.

The really useful thing about sampling distributions is that, if your sample size is large enough (usually at least greater than 30, some say 50), the distribution of the sample means is always normally distributed even if the original population is not (Sullivan, 2008). You can thank the central limit theorem. For the purposes of

this text, you don't need to delve too much into the explanation. The takeaway message is that when a population is not distributed normally, you may need to use other methods to analyze it (see the Appendix for more information on working with small samples B).

TABLE 5-1	Sampling Distribution for the Mean Age of Nurses
Sample	**Mean Age**
One	28
Two	30
Three	30
Four	30
Five	28
Six	26
Seven	32
Eight	32
Nine	34

FIGURE 5-1	Graph of Sample Distribution of Mean Age from Nine Samples.

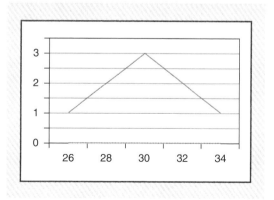

FROM THE STATISTICIAN *Brendan Heavey*

The Central Limit Theorem and Standardized Scores

The central limit theorem is your friend. It makes a lot of analyses a lot simpler. It is a little tough to grasp, perhaps, but if you apply yourself just a little bit, you will be able to pick it up without a problem. Then you can apply it later anytime you want.

One way to understand the central limit theorem is to see what happens when you roll a bunch of 10-sided dice. You can apply this analogy to any random experiment that involves identically likely outcomes.

If you were to roll a 10-sided die 1,000 times and plot a histogram of your results, the graph could look something like the one in **Figure 5-2**. You could get a huge amount of possible bar charts, but they would all look something like the one in the figure. In fact, in the long run, this experiment would use what we call the *uniform distribution* because all cases are equally likely. If we were to roll a single die 1,000, 2,000, or even 10,000 times, all the bars would still look approximately the same.

Now let's think about what would happen if you were to use two 10-sided dice, roll them 1,000 times, and calculate the average value shown on the faces. It just so happens I enjoy doing this sort of thing in my spare time, so I went ahead and did so. The result is shown in **Figure 5-3**. What do you notice? The bars tend to look more bell shaped, don't they? There were a

FIGURE 5-2   **Central Limit Theorem: One 10-Sided Die Rolled 1,000 Times.**

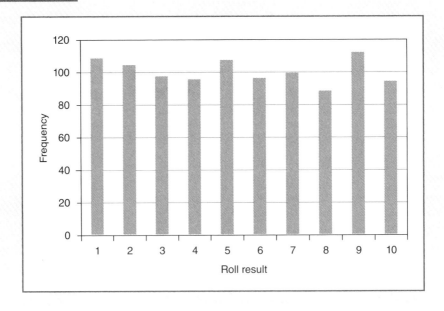

| FIGURE 5-3 | **Central Limit Theorem: Two 10-Sided Dice Rolled 1,000 Times and Averaged.** |

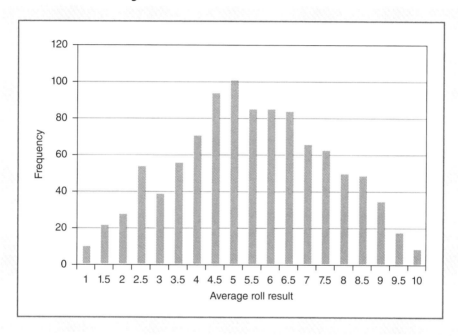

whole lot more results between 4 and 6 than there were 1s and 10s. When you roll two dice, there are a lot more ways to get an average between 4 and 6 than there are to get a 1 or a 10. In fact, the only way to average a 1 is by having both dice come up with 1s.

Now let's look at what happens when you use six 10-sided dice and take the average. The bar graph in **Figure 5-4** looks even more bell shaped.

This progression demonstrates the central limit theorem. In fact, what the underlying distributions look like doesn't matter; you could use a 4-sided die, a 12-sided die, a 6-sided die, or a 20-sided die and plot the outcomes. As you take more and more samples, the resulting distribution of the averages of all the dice will tend to look more and more bell shaped.

Remember that we're talking about the mean value of all the rolls. You can't just roll a single die a million times and expect it to look more and more bell shaped as you increase the number of rolls. You have to look at the mean value across multiple experiments.

(continues)

FROM THE STATISTICIAN *Brendan Heavey*

FIGURE 5-4   **Central Limit Theorem: Six 10-Sided Dice Rolled 1,000 Times and Averaged.**

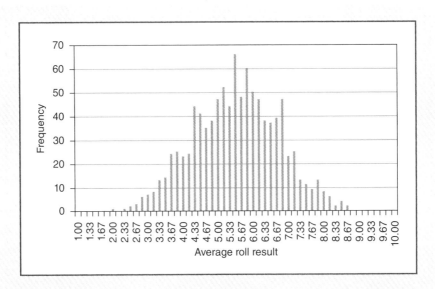

The central limit theorem is one of the most important in all of statistics. It can be proven, but it takes a whole lot of math that I'm sure you don't want to see. You can make some very important and very interesting deductions from this theorem, however. One is that when you take a sample in any experiment, the population variables can be distributed in any manner you want, but the mean of the sample measurement will always be distributed as a normal distribution in the long run. This becomes really important when you compare the means of two samples. (Curb your enthusiasm! I know I can't wait!)

NONPROBABILITY SAMPLING

The reality of research is that it has budgetary and time limits. In these situations, sometimes nonprobability sampling methods are necessary or simply more practical. **Nonprobability sampling** consists of methods in which subjects do *not* have the same chance of being selected for participation; it is *not randomized*. When you are reading nursing research, never assume a sample was randomly selected. You need to identify how the sample was selected before you can tell whether the claims that the researcher makes are valid or what their limitations may be.

Types of Nonprobability Sampling

Nonprobability sampling can be used in many different ways in both quantitative and qualitative research. Two of the most popular methods for quantitative research are convenience sampling and quota sampling, whereas qualitative research may employ network sampling or purposive sampling.

Convenience Sampling

The most popular form of nonprobability sampling in healthcare research is **convenience sampling**, which is simply collecting data from the available group. For example, suppose you were trying to determine the mean age of the nurses in your hospital. You go to the oncology unit and ask all the nurses working that shift their age. You would be taking a convenience sample. Convenience samples are usually relatively quick and inexpensive, but they may not be representative of the population and therefore may limit any inferences you may choose to make about the population.

Quota Sampling

In **quota sampling**, you select the proportions of the sample for different subgroups, as in stratified sampling. For example, if 50% of your population works the day shift, 30% works the evening shift, and 20% works the night shift, your sample will have those same proportions. I bet right now you are thinking, "But this doesn't seem to be different from stratified random sampling." Well, so far, you are right; nothing is different yet. The difference is after this point. Remember, if you need a final sample size of 100, with stratified random sampling, you would *randomly* select 50 subjects from day shift workers, 30 from evening shift workers,

and 20 from night shift workers. Quota sampling, on the other hand, is nonprobability sampling, so it is *not* randomized. After you decide on the proportions of the sample, you collect subjects continuously until you have 50 day shift subjects, 30 evening shift subjects, and 20 night shift subjects.

Now suppose that you decide to collect the quota sample at 3:30 in the lobby of your hospital. Everyone who participates gets a free coffee coupon. Fifty day shift nurses participate on their way out, and 30 evening shift nurses participate on their way in. You have enrolled all your day and evening nurses but are still waiting for the night nurses. At 10:45 the night shift nurses start to come through the lobby. As you are surveying the night shift staffers, an evening nurse, ending her shift, comes over and volunteers to participate. You cannot include her because you already have your quota of evening shift nurses and are still collecting only night shift nurses. The evening shift nurse becomes irate because she really wants to be in your study (read "really wants the coffee"), and she calls several of her friends to come in and volunteer. (Nurses *will* do a lot for free coffee.) They, too, are upset because they were not working that day and were therefore never given the opportunity to participate. Because they worked the day and evening shifts, they are also not eligible to participate because you have already filled the quotas for these shifts.

You end up sitting in the lobby with several very upset day and evening nurses who don't understand why you can't let them participate, at the same time still asking the night shift nurses to join the study and giving them coffee. "The night shift gets everything!" the other nurses complain. Because you are exceptionally patient and have already had your extra coffee that day, you patiently explain that quota sampling does not give the same opportunity to everyone to participate. You are very sorry. You would love to give everyone free coffee, but you need only night nurses now. This is how quota sampling works. Once you have reached the quota for that particular group, no matter how many more subjects from that group arrive, you do not enroll them and collect data only from the groups for which you have not met your quota.

Of course, after such a stressful experience, you may also decide either to change your sampling method or to go to a different hospital to collect data next time. These nurses are intense!

NONPROBABILITY SAMPLING IN QUALITATIVE RESEARCH

Many other nonprobability-based sampling methods are used more frequently with qualitative research. Network sampling, for example, utilizes the social networks of friends and families to gather information. This technique is frequently used when you need information about groups that hesitate to participate in research, such as youth gangs. Another technique, purposive sampling, includes subjects because they have particularly strong bases of information. You may decide to use network sampling to study youth gangs after you are able to gain the trust and support of a gang leader. She then refers other members of her gang to you, and you are able eventually to speak to a group of 10 youth gang members. You may then decide to collect a purposive sample (specific individuals are selected to participate because of the information they are able to contribute) and further study three of these young women because they are lifelong gang members and can give you the greatest insight into the characteristics and behaviors you are studying.

INCLUSION AND EXCLUSION CRITERIA

No matter which sampling method you select, as the researcher you need to develop sample inclusion and exclusion criteria.

- **Inclusion criteria** make up the list of characteristics a subject must have to be eligible to participate in your study. These criteria identify the target population and limit the generalizability of your study results to this population. For example, if you are studying the effect of taking a multivitamin on future prostate cancer development, the foremost inclusion criterion is male gender. (Only men have prostates, so it would be pointless to include women in this study.)
- **Exclusion criteria** are the criteria or characteristics that eliminate a subject from being eligible to participate in your study. Exclusion criteria frequently include the current or past presence of the outcome of interest. For example, in your study about the vitamin-mediated prevention of prostate cancer, having prostate cancer would be one of your exclusion criteria. If the subject already has or has had the disease, you can't determine whether the vitamin helps to prevent it.

SAMPLE SIZE

We are going to spend some more time talking in detail about sample size in Chapter 7, but it is important to note that our sample collection method is only one aspect of ensuring we gather the information we are seeking in a study. Another critical piece is collecting the correct number of subjects for the purposes of your study. The larger your study, the better you will be able to find a difference that really exists. This is sometimes referred to as the power of a study. Larger samples make more powerful studies. Of course, larger samples cost more and can have other complicating factors, but generally speaking, researchers aim to enroll as many subjects as possible under the circumstances.

Summary

That was a lot of information to take in for one chapter, so take a deep breath and allow your brain to slow down. Let's highlight the main ideas.

A sampling method consists of the processes that help you pick the subjects for your sample from the population you are interested in studying. The two main kinds of sampling methods are probability sampling and nonprobability sampling. Probability sampling involves techniques in which the probability of selecting each subject is known; thus, subjects are selected randomly. Types of probability sampling include simple random sampling, systematic sampling, stratified sampling, and cluster sampling. Nonprobability sampling involves methods in which subjects do not have the same chance of being selected for participation. In other words, sampling is not randomized. Nonprobability sampling includes convenience sampling, quota sampling, network sampling, and purposive sampling.

When you are collecting samples, sampling error can occur; that is, some differences between the sample and the population should be expected to occur due to randomization or chance. Sampling bias can also occur, however; it is the result of a systematic error in the sample selection, rendering it nongeneralizable to the original population.

Finally, all research studies have inclusion and exclusion criteria. Inclusion criteria are characteristics that a subject must have to participate in your study. Exclusion criteria are the criteria or characteristics that eliminate a subject from being eligible to participate.

You are done with this chapter. Take a break. Drink some tea and unwind a bit. You've earned a break!

CHAPTER 5 REVIEW QUESTIONS

1. What is the difference between probability and nonprobability sampling?

2. Identify whether probability or nonprobability sampling is utilized for each entry in the following list:
   - Convenience sampling
   - Cluster sampling
   - Simple random sampling
   - Quota sampling
   - Systematic sampling
   - Stratified sampling

3. What is the difference between sampling error and sampling bias? Which one is very concerning to researchers?

Research Application

Questions 4–5: One study used a convenience sample drawn from clients utilizing two community-based obstetric offices in an area with lower socioeconomic status. The sample was drawn largely from the community surrounding the offices, and the findings may not be generalizable to this population or other populations that differ significantly from this sample.*

4. Why should a reader be careful about developing inferences about the population of interest from the article?

5. How could the researcher have designed this study differently so that developing inferences about the population of interest would be less of a concern?

6. Hemoglobin levels are usually 12–16 g/100 mL for women and 14–18 g/100 mL for men. If you have a sampling distribution of mean hemoglobin levels (collected from 60 hospitals) with a mean of 16 g/100 mL and a standard deviation of 2 g/100 mL, calculate the range of hemoglobin levels that would include 68% of your sample means.

7. What percentage of sample means would fall between 12 g/100 mL and 20 g/100 mL?

8. If one of the hospitals in your sample was a Veterans Affairs facility with 97% male patients, would you expect the mean hemoglobin level collected only from the patients at that hospital to be any different from those of other hospitals?

9. If one of the hospitals in your sample was the regional Women's and Children's Hospital, would you expect the mean hemoglobin level collected at that hospital to be different from that of the other hospitals?

10. You would like to compare the wait time at your clinic this year versus last year. Your electronic medical record database contains the check-in time and rooming time for all patients seen in the last 2 years. You import the data into your SPSS statistics program and program the computer to select randomly 500 patients seen last year and 500 patients seen this year. What type of sample is this? Is it a probability or nonprobability sampling method?

11. You decide to start again comparing the wait time at your clinic this year versus last year, this time programing SPSS to select every 14th patient each year. What type of sample is this? Is it a probability or nonprobability sample?

*This text is reprinted with the permission of Elsevier and was originally published in Heavey, E., Moysich, K., Hyland, A., Druschel, C., & Sill, M. (2008). Female adolescents' perception of male partners' pregnancy desire. *Journal of Midwifery and Women's Health, 53*(4), 338–344. Copyright Elsevier (2008).

12. A researcher examining drinking patterns in his county distributes his survey at a bar on the first Friday of three consecutive months. What type of sample is this? Is it a probability or nonprobability sample?

13. The researcher in Review Question 12 decides that he wants his sample of 200 to be 50% female and distributes his survey at the bar to the first 100 women who arrive and the first 100 men who arrive. This is what type of sample? Is it a probability or nonprobability sample?

14. You would like to know the average wait time of adult patients seen in federally funded health clinics in the United States. You randomly select 100 clinics and then collect the wait time for 100 randomly selected patient visits. What type of sample is this? Is it a probability or nonprobability sample?

15. You conduct a well-designed study involving a random sample. Your analysis shows this sample is normally distributed and representative of the population; however, the mean age in the sample is 29.4 years, and the mean age in the population is 30 years. What is this type of difference called, and what is the likely cause of the difference? Should the researcher be concerned?

16. A researcher wants to examine drinking patterns in men and women in bars in New York State. She randomly selects five bars and then randomly selects subjects at those bars to complete her surveys on four randomly selected weekends. However, she did not realize that two of the five bars selected were for gay men, and another bar was having a draft special for the football playoff games for three of the four weekends. Her sample ends up being 85% male, but the population who attends bars is only 65% male. Is this sample representative? Why or why not? Would this be an example of sample error or sample bias? Should the researcher be concerned?

Questions 17–20: You would like to ensure that your sample is representative of the racial mix seen in your population of interest. The population is 50% Asian, 20% African American, 20% Caucasian, and 10% other. You need a sample of 500 subjects. You program SPSS to select randomly 250 Asian subjects from your population, 100 African American subjects, 100 Caucasian subjects, and 50 subjects identified as other.

17. What type of sample is this? Is it a probability or nonprobability sample?

18. You are interested in how race may affect total cholesterol. Your study classifies race in the categories described above. What level of measurement is this variable?

19. What is your dependent variable?

20. Your sample is normally distributed with an average total cholesterol of 211 and a standard deviation of 7. In what range would you expect the total cholesterol to be for 68% of your sample?

Questions 21–25: A nurse researcher is studying the impact of social media usage on the quality of adolescent relationships. She identifies 22 teen subjects and asks about whom they contact on Facebook, via Twitter, and via text messaging. She then follows up with an interview with those who have the most contacts and examines these relationships further.

21. What is the independent variable in this study?

22. What is the dependent variable in this study?

23. If the quality of adolescent relationships is reported as poor, good, or excellent, what level variable is this?

24. Instead, the researcher asks these adolescents to rank the quality of their relationships on a scale of 0–10. What level of measurement would this variable be?

25. What type of sampling method is this? Is it probability or nonprobability sampling?

Questions 26–30: You conduct a well-designed study involving a random sample ($n = 84$). Age is measured in years. Your analysis shows that in this sample, age is normally distributed and representative of the population. The youngest subjects are 15 ($n = 2$), one subject is 16, and the oldest subject is 46 years old; the mean age is 29.4 years, and there is a standard deviation of 3 years.

26. What is the median age in this sample?

27. What age range would include 95% of the subjects in your sample?

28. What is the age range of the sample?

29. What percentage of your sample is 15 years of age or less?

30. If age is measured as 15–20 years, 25–35 years, and 35 years, what level of measurement is this variable?

31. If a variable is measured as eligible to vote and not eligible to vote, what level of measurement is this variable?

32. If you randomly select 250 individuals who are on a voter registration list and 72 report they will vote for an independent candidate, what percentage is planning to vote for an independent candidate?

Questions 33–35: You decide to interview all college athletic team captains at three state universities because of their direct knowledge of team initiation activities and hazing practices.

33. What type of sample is this? Is it a probability or nonprobability sampling method?

34. Your subjects must have been team captains for at least 3 months, on a Division I university–affiliated sports team, who are eligible to play in the upcoming season. These subject characteristics are examples of what?

35. Team captains currently on the injured or inactive list are not eligible to participate in the study. This is an example of what?

36. A study examined the average daily activity level of children. Three observers recorded the activity level of 15 children each during the month of February in upstate New York. The children were all 6 to 9 years old. The observers reported that children are physically active for only 38 minutes a day (on average) and concluded that a public health intervention to increase the activity level of children was needed. What factors might concern you about this study and the researchers' conclusion?

37. The observations in Review Questions 36 were all made between 10 a.m. and 3 p.m. on Mondays, Wednesdays, and Fridays. Do you think that is important to report in the study? Why? How might this information affect the results?

ANSWERS TO ODD-NUMBERED CHAPTER 5 REVIEW QUESTIONS

1. With probability sampling, the probability of selecting each subject is known and is the same. With nonprobability sampling, the subjects do not have the same chance of being selected.

3. Sampling error is random error due to chance. Systematic error results in a nonrandom sample and is very concerning to researchers.

5. A randomized sample improves representativeness and expands generalizability.

7. 95% (mean 16 ± 2 standard deviations)

9. Yes, hemoglobin levels are lower for women and children.

11. Systematic sample, probability sample

13. Convenience sample with quota sampling, nonprobability

15. A sampling error likely due to chance or randomization; the researcher does not have to be concerned.

17. Stratified, probability sample

19. Total cholesterol

21. Social media use

23. Ordinal

25. Network sampling, nonprobability

27. 23.4–35.4 years

29. 2/84 = 2.4%

31. Nominal

33. Purposeful sample, nonprobability sampling

35. Exclusion criteria

37. Yes, most children in the age group would be in school during this time and may not have the opportunity to be physically active until after they are done with school, which could bias the results; students' schedules may differ on Mondays, Wednesdays, and Fridays from the rest of the week; and so on.

GENERATING THE RESEARCH IDEA

WHAT IS MY RESEARCH IDEA?

OBJECTIVES

By the end of this chapter students will be able to:

- State the null hypothesis.
- Define an alternative hypothesis.
- Describe hypothesis testing.
- Compare rejecting the null hypothesis and failing to reject the null hypothesis.
- Correlate alpha, the chance of a type one error, and statistical significance.
- Identify a type one error, and propose one method to avoid it.

- Distinguish between statistically significant results and nonsignificant results in a current research article.
- Debate clinical significance given a research article with statistical significance present.
- Analyze statistical information to determine whether statistical significance is present.

KEY TERMS

Alpha (α)
The significance level, usually 0.05. The probability of incorrectly rejecting the null hypothesis or making a type one error.

Alternative hypothesis
Usually the relationship or association or difference that the researcher actually believes to be present.

Clinically significant
A result that is statistically significant *and* clinically useful.

Fail to reject the null hypothesis
Not having enough statistical strength to show a difference or an association.

Hypothesis
An observation or idea that can be tested.

Hypothesis testing
The application of a statistical test to determine whether an observation or idea is to be refuted or accepted.

Null hypothesis
No difference or association between variables that is any greater or less than would be expected by chance.

Reject the null hypothesis
Having enough statistical strength to show a difference or an association.

Statistical significance
The difference observed between two samples is large enough to conclude that it is not simply due to chance.

Type one error
Incorrectly rejecting the null hypothesis.

HYPOTHESIS TESTING

When you arrive at the clinic at 8 a.m., you are prepared to administer the flu vaccine to patients who show up for one. Already people are waiting, and many are wearing business attire. The turnout is much higher than your clinic expected, processing everyone is taking longer than expected, and you are the only nurse. The patients are brought into a central receiving area, their background information is collected, and then they come to your station for the actual injection. After the first hour, you notice that most of your patients are elderly or unemployed. You realize that it is after now after 9 a.m. Very few individuals who report outside employment arrive during the hours of 9 a.m. and 5 p.m. You start to wonder whether employed individuals are less likely to get their flu shots because they are unable to come to the clinic during standard business hours, and those who arrived before work may not have been able to stay due to the long delays.

This is a **hypothesis**, an observation or idea that can be tested. You decide to determine whether your observation is actually true. First, you develop your **null hypothesis**, which states that there is no difference or association between variables that is any greater or less than would be expected by chance. (The null hypothesis is represented as H_0.) In this case, the null hypothesis is that there is no relationship between employment status and having a flu shot at your clinic. The **alternative hypothesis** is usually the relationship, association, or difference that the researcher actually believes to be present. (The alternative hypothesis is represented as H_1.) In this case, your alternative hypothesis is that those who are employed are less likely to get a flu shot at your clinic. **Hypothesis testing**, a fancy term for figuring out whether you are right, involves using a statistical test to determine whether your hypothesis is true. In this case, when the clinic closes that first night, you decide to collect the information that was gathered on all the patients who arrived at the clinic from 8 a.m. until 9 p.m. that week. This is your sample.

Your statistical analysis of the sample enables you to do one of two things:

- If the trend of having very few employed patients arriving for flu shots at your clinic continued throughout the day, you may find a statistically significant difference (we'll tell you how to do this later in the chapter) between the number of employed people who received the flu shot at your clinic that week and those who were not employed. You are then in a position to **reject the null hypothesis**. You have determined the difference between the two groups is greater than the difference you might expect to result from chance. You have evidence of a statistically significant relationship between employment status and receiving a flu shot at your clinic, and you have demonstrated support for your alternative hypothesis.
- On the other hand, let's say that you collect and analyze the data from the whole week and find that although there were fewer employed people receiving flu shots

between 9 a.m. and 5 p.m. (your initial impression), between 8 a.m. and 9 a.m. and between 5 p.m. and 9 p.m., most of the flu shot recipients were employed. In this case, your statistical analysis may not show a significant difference between the number of people who received the flu shot who were employed and those who were not. You would then **fail to reject the null hypothesis**. This is the important point: You can never "accept" or "prove" the null hypothesis, which is the absence of something. You can only "disprove" it (reject it) or "fail to disprove" it (fail to reject it).

Obstetrics nurses usually understand this slightly confusing concept fairly quickly, so let's use their clinical experience to create an analogy and help you, too. When a pregnant patient has an ultrasound, the technician attempts to determine the sex of the infant by detecting the presence of a penis. The null hypothesis is that there is no penis. The alternative hypothesis is that there is one. If a penis is detected, the ultrasound technician can state that there is one and that the baby is a boy. If a penis is not detected, the technician cannot be sure that there isn't one; it might be present but undetected (Corty, 2007). As a nurse–midwife, I frequently explain to my patients that if the ultrasound technician told them they are carrying a baby boy, they could consider the report fairly reliable (but notice this is still not a probability of 100%). However, I have been in the delivery room when a predicted girl turned out to be a bashful boy. Never overstate what your data allows you to say! You can never say for sure that something does not exist, but the mere presence of what you are looking for can demonstrate that it does. It is also important to remember that statistics is all about probability, and there is always a possibility of an error, so you can never "prove" anything with absolute certainty. The technician who thinks she sees a baby boy could still be wrong.

STATISTICAL SIGNIFICANCE

Statistical significance means that the difference you observe between two samples is large enough to conclude that it is not simply due to chance. Statistical significance can be shown in many different ways, but the basic idea remains the same: If you take two or more representative samples from the same population, you would expect to find approximately the same difference again and again. If you have a statistically significant result, you can reject the null hypothesis.

But how do you know whether your result is statistically significant? At the beginning of the study, the researcher selects the significance level, or **alpha**, which is usually 0.05. This number is simply the probability assigned to incorrectly rejecting the null hypothesis, or to making what is called a **type one error**. For example, you conduct a study examining the association between eating a high-fiber breakfast and 10 a.m. serum glucose levels. The null hypothesis is that a high-fiber breakfast is not associated with the 10 a.m. serum glucose levels. The alternative is that it is. You select an alpha of 0.05, which means you are willing to accept that there is a 5% chance that you will reject the null hypothesis incorrectly and report that eating a high-fiber breakfast is associated with a change in blood sugar levels at 10 a.m. when in actuality it is not.

The alpha is therefore the preestablished limit on the chance the researcher is willing to take that he or she will report a statistically significant difference that does not exist. The researcher is willing to report that a statistically significant difference exists right up until the point when the probability of being incorrect is about 5% (alpha = 0.05). An alpha of 0.05 can also be interpreted to mean that the researcher is 95% sure that the significant difference that he or she is reporting is correct.

Think about this in terms of waking a provider in the middle of the night. You are willing to do that if you are 95% sure your patient has an immediate concern, but you are not so willing to do that if you are only 15% sure that your patient has a pressing issue. The ramifications of being wrong can be substantial at 3 a.m. no matter what you decide, so you may make the call, or you may continue to gather more observations until you are more certain. Remember, all statistical test results are reported as probabilities. No one is absolutely certain that they are correct!

Corresponding to the alpha (which is represented by α) is what statisticians call the p-value. Remember that we started to talk about this concept in Chapter 3. The p-value is the probability of observing a value of a test statistic if the null hypothesis (there is no relationship, association, or difference between the variables) is true. In other words, a p-value tells you the probability of finding your test statistic if there is no relationship between the variables. This is also the probability that an observed relationship, association, or difference is due simply to chance. For example, if your study examining the consumption of a high-fiber breakfast and 10 a.m. glucose levels has a test statistic with a p-value of 0.03, then the probability that the observations in your study would occur if there were no relationship between these variables (or by chance) is only 3%. This means that you are 97% sure the variables in your study do have a relationship.

If your study has an alpha of 0.05, it means you are willing to accept up to a 5% chance of making a type one error and reporting that a relationship exists when it is just by chance. If the actual *p*-value of your test statistic shows you have only a 3% chance of making a type one error ($p = 0.03$), then you are within error limits that are comfortable for you (5% or less) and can confidently reject the null hypothesis. Rejecting the null hypothesis means that you report a relationship, an association, or a difference between the variables.

So now you know that if the *p*-value is less than the alpha, you should reject the null hypothesis. However, if the *p*-value is greater than the alpha, the chance of making a type one error is greater than the level you are comfortable with, and you should fail to reject the null hypothesis. In this case ($p >$ alpha), you would fail to reject the null hypothesis and report that there is no relationship, association, or difference between the variables.

Subtracting the *p*-value from 1 tells you how sure the researcher is about rejecting the null hypothesis. For example, a *p*-value of 0.03 means the researcher is 97% sure that the observed relationship is not just due to chance. Sometimes thinking of it this way helps.

| FIGURE 6-1 | *p* < alpha. |

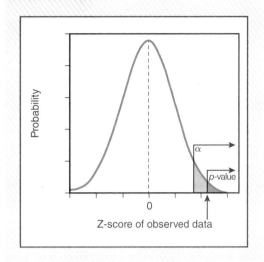

You can see how this looks on the probability distribution in **Figure 6-1**. A low *p*-value is way out in the tail of the probability distribution. If it is smaller than your alpha value, then the probability of finding this test result if the null hypothesis is true is smaller than the chance you are willing to take of being incorrect about rejecting the null. This is a graphic illustration of *p* < alpha, which means you have statistically significant results and should reject the null hypothesis.

FROM THE STATISTICIAN *Brendan Heavey*

Alpha of 0.05: Standard Convention versus Experiment Specific

Interpreting *p*-values can be a science in and of itself. Let me share with you how I think of *p*-values.

Think about your favorite courtroom drama. Whether you recall O. J. Simpson's trial, *A Few Good Men*, *To Kill a Mockingbird*, or *Erin Brockovich*, the defendants are innocent until proven guilty in all these situations. Therefore, the null

(continues)

FROM THE STATISTICIAN *Brendan Heavey*

hypothesis in these "experiments" is that the defendant is innocent. At all these trials, a defendant is declared not guilty, never innocent. The trial is being conducted—like an experiment—to determine whether to reject the null hypothesis. The null hypothesis cannot be proven; it can only be disproven.

In O. J.'s case, a lot of people thought there was enough evidence to reject the null hypothesis of innocence and find him guilty. However, as in any criminal case, O. J. had to be declared guilty beyond a reasonable doubt. This is a very stringent criterion. Later, in the civil case, the district attorney only had to show a preponderance of evidence to have him declared liable, which was a much easier task. So O. J. was found not guilty in the criminal trial but liable in the civil trial. This split decision is the equivalent of different alpha levels determining statistical significance in statistical experiments. The courts reduced the stringency of the test from determining criminal guilt to civil liability by reducing the burden of proof necessary to reject the null hypothesis between the two tests. Scientists can do the same thing in statistical tests by increasing alpha (which "decreases the burden of proof" in your study). Notice that showing a defendant is liable in a civil trial (due to a preponderance of evidence) is easier to do than showing he or she is guilty in a criminal trial (beyond a reasonable doubt). Think of a statistical test the same way. If your *p*-value is 0.07, you would reject the null hypothesis if your alpha is 0.10 (less stringent) but not if your alpha is 0.05 (more stringent). It is easier to reject the null hypothesis at the 0.10 level than the 0.05 level.

Note that 0.05 is a very arbitrary alpha cutoff. It has persisted to this day only because R. A. Fisher preferred it, and he's one of the most important statisticians and scientists of all time. He started the practice back in the 1920s, and it has stuck ever since. However, at times, scientists use a more stringent cutoff of 0.01 or a less stringent one of 0.1. Determining statistical significance is a sliding scale, just like the sliding scale of burden of proof in the courtroom.

I would like to thank Jeffrey J. Isaacson, J. D., Professor at Emmanuel College, for taking the time to clarify the terminology utilized in civil trial procedures.

STATISTICAL SIGNIFICANCE VERSUS CLINICAL SIGNIFICANCE

Statistically significant differences are not the same as **clinically significant** differences. Clinically significant differences are large enough to indicate a preferential course of treatment or a difference in clinical approach to patient care. To be clinically significant, a result must be statistically significant *and* clinically useful. Results that are statistically significant are not necessarily clinically significant, which is a more subjective conclusion.

For example, as a nurse manager, you are approached by the largest chocolate sales team in your region. They say that the newest research shows that patients who receive free chocolate from the hospital are discharged earlier. Well, you might be interested in reading the study. The chocolate team conducted a study with 700,000 participants and found that those who were given free chocolate went home on average 2 minutes earlier than those who didn't. Although you know chocolate makes people feel better, you do not see these statistically significant results as being

FROM THE STATISTICIAN *Brendan Heavey*

Statistical Testing

What if we want to use the information we collect to make informed decisions? What if we want to use the data to decide how to treat patients or how to predict who will most benefit from new treatments? Questions like these make up the core of hypothesis testing. This "From the Statistician" feature is a little more difficult, but it is at the very heart of the statistical science presented in this text, so try to hang in there with me.

Most statistical testing procedures can be broken down into the five steps shown in **Figure 6-2**. A hypothesis test is like a funnel that sorts a whole bunch of information in the form of sample data and decision rules, and then spits out a single, easy-to-understand *p*-value. Isn't it great that there is an easy-to-understand answer after all that work!

- State the null and alternative hypotheses.
- *Significance level:* Determine which alpha to use to determine statistical significance.
- *Statistical test:* Determine which statistical test to use.
- Compare the distribution of the statistic computed in step 3 to the distribution under the null hypothesis, and report a *p*-value.
- *Decision rule:* Decide whether or not to reject the null hypothesis. (Is the sample distribution different enough from the null distribution to say it is more than a chance occurrence?)

| FIGURE 6-2 | **Hypothesis Testing Steps.** |

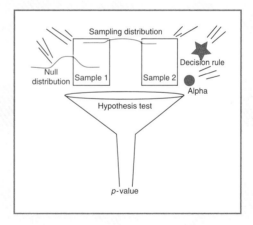

clinically significant because a saving of 2 minutes has very little impact on your unit. Besides, what do the follow-up studies say about tooth decay? In addition, having a very large sample size (700,000 people) in a study might result in statistical significance even though the difference found (the effect size) is actually very small.

HYPOTHESIS TESTING IN ACTION

Let's take it from the top and go step-by-step through hypothesis testing. The first two steps in a hypothesis test are relatively straightforward, and you already know how to do them. First, you state your null and alternative hypotheses; then you pick the significance level (alpha) that you wish to have in your study. Remember that, typically, the alpha is 0.05, which means that if you find a difference, you are 95% sure it is truly there, not just a chance occurrence.

You also already know that the *p*-value is going to be compared to the alpha. It is just a probability statement about the actual research results. Just as probability ranges between 0 and 1, so do *p*-values. The closer a *p*-value gets to 1, the more likely the related event is (in this case, the conclusion). The closer the *p*-value gets to 0, the less likely it is. Piece of cake, right?

Choosing which statistical test to perform is more difficult. Which test you choose depends on a number of things, but usually the most important are how many samples will be compared, how many parts of the population will be estimated, and the format of the variables. We will be talking about all different statistical tests in the upcoming chapters, but they have a lot in common, so for now we will speak about them in general terms.

Many tests involve computing a so-called test statistic. One type of test statistic is a *Z*-score, which is probably all coming back to you from Chapter 3. A *Z*-score is simply a test statistic that is a standardized measure in a normal distribution. A *Z*-score tells you how many standard deviations the observation is from the mean. For example, if $Z = 3.4$, the observation is 3.4 standard deviations above the mean score. If $Z = -0.2$, then the observation is 0.2 standard deviations below the mean score. A *Z*-score, like any other test statistic you compute, has a corresponding *p*-value, which is then used to make the decision to reject or fail to reject the null hypothesis. All test statistics you compute have a corresponding probability or *p*-value.

HOW DOES THE TEST STATISTIC COMPARE TO THE NULL HYPOTHESIS?

Let's look at those *p*-values graphically again. **Figure 6-3** is a picture of a hypothesis test using the normal distribution. We can see that the area under the normal curve varies when drawing vertical lines at different *Z*-scores. This area is what we need to know in order to report *p*-values. In this case, 2.5% of the probability can be found in each tail of the distribution. (This is how your alpha is distributed when you have a two-tailed test, which involves a nondirectional alternative hypothesis. For example, when the researcher believes there is a relationship between the independent variable and the dependent variable but isn't sure if the change in the independent variable will be associated with an increase or decrease the

| FIGURE 6-3 | **The Normal Curve.** |

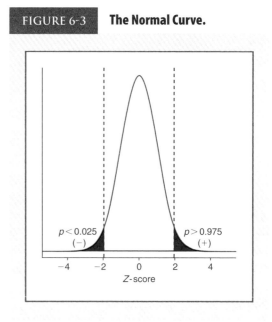

dependent variable.) The area underneath the normal curve, above the horizontal axis, and to the outside of our vertical lines totals 0.05, which is your alpha value (0.025 in each tail). These vertical lines also represent the Z-value that corresponds with these probability levels. A Z-score of 1.96 corresponds to an alpha of 0.05 in a normal distribution. In this case, the test statistic you computed was a Z-value of 2, which is greater than 1.96 (the cutoff for statistical significance on the horizontal axis), so our statistical test falls further out into the upper tail of the null distribution. Whenever that happens, we say that the observed data is significantly different from what we would expect under the null distribution (or if the null distribution were true).

This should make sense conceptually. As your observations get farther and farther away from the center of the data (mean), two things happen:

- The Z-score (test statistic) gets pushed farther and farther into the tails of the statistical distribution.
- The p-value associated with that Z-score (test statistic) gets smaller and smaller.

And, as you already know, the smaller the p-value is, the less likely it is that this observation is due simply to chance and the more sure you can be that the difference you found is actually there.

APPLYING THE DECISION RULE

To apply our decision rule, we need to see if our p-value is less than or greater than alpha. In our last example, the probability of observing the statistical results we found if the null hypothesis were true (p-value) is low and in this case less than alpha. Because $p <$ alpha,

we conclude this observed difference is not just due to sampling error or chance; we reject the null hypothesis and report that a difference, association, or relationship exists between the two variables. If the p-value were greater than alpha, our decision would be to fail to reject the null and report that there is no relationship, association, or difference between the variables.

TEST STATISTICS AND CORRESPONDING P-VALUES

Whew! That was a tough one, but you should now be starting to understand the link between test statistics and p-values. This concept directly transfers from Z-scores to other test statistics such as T-scores, F-scores, and chi-squared scores. All of the calculated test statistics have a corresponding p-value, which is what you have to look at to determine if there is a statistically significant difference and what conclusion you should draw about the null hypothesis. The different tests differ in the types of data involved as well as in the quantities being estimated, but they work on this same principle. If the p-value associated with the computed test statistic is less than the alpha value chosen in the decision rule, we should reject the null hypothesis.

SUMMARY

You have just completed Chapter 6! The concepts are getting more technical, but keep reviewing and practicing to maintain and enhance your knowledge. Now we can review some of the important concepts in this chapter.

A hypothesis is an observation or idea that can be tested. The null hypothesis states that there is no relationship, association, or difference. The alternative hypothesis is the opposite of the null: There is a relationship, association, or difference (what you actually think is true). Hypothesis testing involves using a sample to determine whether your hypothesis is true.

When you reject the null hypothesis, you have found statistical support for your alternative hypothesis. When you fail to reject the null hypothesis, you do not have enough statistical strength to say there is a relationship or an association. There may not really be a relationship, or you may not have a sample that is large enough. You can never accept the null hypothesis. If you reject the null hypothesis incorrectly, it is a type one error.

Statistical significance means that the difference you observed between two samples is large enough that it is not simply due to chance. To determine statistical significance, you need to identify a significance level, called the alpha, which is usually 0.05. If your p-value is less than alpha, you have statistical significance. For something to be clinically significant, a result must be statistically significant and clinically useful.

This chapter presented a lot of information, but if you are able to grasp these concepts, you are doing well! If it still seems a bit murky, don't worry. We will continue to work with these ideas and reinforce them as you build your knowledge!

CHAPTER 6 REVIEW QUESTIONS

1. For review questions 1–5, you are conducting a study to determine whether there is an association between years worked in nursing and salary earned. Write the null and alternative hypotheses.

2. If you find a p-value of 0.09, what would you conclude?

3. If you find a p-value of 0.03, what would you conclude?

4. If you reject the null hypothesis, what type of error is it if you are wrong?

5. If your p-value is 0.03, is the conclusion clinically significant?

6. For review questions 6–15, you are conducting a study to determine whether there is an association between a positive toxicology screen for Rohypnol (flunitrazepam) and signs of sexual assault in a sample collected from three large emergency rooms throughout your state. Write the null and alternative hypotheses.

7. As the primary investigator in this study, you realize your results may be utilized in a courtroom setting, and you do not want to make a type one error. Would you prefer an alpha of 0.05, 0.10, or 0.01?

8. Your study includes all individuals who arrive in the three emergency rooms with a diagnosis of sexual assault over a 1-month period. This is what type of sample?

9. You conduct the study with an alpha of 0.05, and your test statistic has a *p*-value of 0.02. What do you conclude?

10. You get the consent of the study participants and conduct a follow-up study in which you interview the family members of the individuals included in your study. This is an example of what type of sampling?

11. You ask the family members to describe the appearance and the manner of the individuals who were assaulted when they were taken to the emergency room. Is this a qualitative or quantitative measurement?

12. You also collect a measure of the patient's sedation provided by the sexual assault nurse examiner. It is on a 5-point scale: 0 for no sedation, 1 for mild sedation, 2 for moderate sedation, 3 for heavy sedation, and 5 for unable to arouse. What level of measurement is this?

13. In your sample of 45 patients, 10 showed no signs of sedation, 12 were mildly sedated, 3 were moderately sedated, 13 were heavily sedated, and 7 were not arousable. What percentage were mild or moderately sedated?

14. What is the median level of sedation?

15. You are putting together a grouped frequencies table and want to categorize these responses as patients showing signs of sedation and those not showing signs of sedation. How many patients showed signs of sedation? What percentage of your sample is this?

Questions 16–40: A researcher believes there is risk between the strain of human papillomavirus (HPV) infection and the risk of cervical cell abnormalities.

16. Write an appropriate null hypothesis.

17. Write an appropriate alternative hypothesis.

18. If HPV infection is measured as not infected, infected with a low-risk strain, or infected with a high-risk strain, what level of measurement is this variable?

19. If the presence of cervical cell abnormalities is measured as biopsy results positive or negative, what level of measurement is this variable?

20. If cervical cell abnormalities are measured as biopsy pathology results of negative, CIN I, CIN II, CIN III, or cancer in situ (CIS) (these are progressively worse levels of abnormality), what level of measurement is the variable?

21. In the population, 30% of cervical biopsies are negative, 40% are CIN I, 20% are CIN II, 5% are CIN III, and 5% are CIS. A random selection of hospitals is made, and a random selection of biopsy results is reviewed. What type of sample is this?

22. Is it a probability or nonprobability sample?

23. In the random sample of 120 biopsies, 16 are negative, 42 are CIN I, 30 are CIN II, 22 are CIN III, and 10 are CIS. In the same sample, 1 person is HPV negative, 87 are HPV positive with the low-risk strain, and 32 are HPV positive with the high-risk strain. What percentage of your sample is CIN II or greater?

24. What percentage is not infected with a high-risk strain?

25. What percentage has an abnormal cervical biopsy?

26. What is the median biopsy result?

27. What biopsy result is the mode?

28. Can you determine the mean biopsy result? Why or why not?

29. What is the median type of HPV infection?

30. What is the mode for the type of HPV infection?

31. The study reports the association between the type of HPV infection and cervical cell abnormalities has a *p*-value of 0.06. If the alpha for the study is set at 0.05, what should the researcher conclude regarding the null hypothesis? Why?

32. What is the prevalence of HPV infection in this sample?

33. If instead of an alpha of 0.05 the researchers decided to set this pilot study's alpha at 0.10, what would the researcher conclude about the null hypothesis ($p = 0.06$)?

34. If the researcher rejects the null but does so in error, what type of error could he or she be making? What does this type of error mean?

35. If the researcher does find a statistically significant difference, does this mean it is a clinically significant difference?

36. If the researcher reports an alpha of 0.05 and a *p*-value of 0.09, are the results clinically significant? Why or why not?

37. Write what you would conclude about the null hypothesis with the following results at the two different levels of alpha:

Study	*p*-Value	Alpha = 0.05	Alpha = 0.10
A	0.0647		
B	0.912		
C	0.1567		
D	0.0211		
E	0.081		

38. Refer to the table in review question 37. If the researcher is incorrect about the decision made regarding the null hypothesis, which studies could be a type one error at an alpha of 0.05? Why?

39. Refer to the table in review question 37. If the researcher is incorrect about the decision made regarding the null hypothesis, which studies could be a type one error at an alpha of 0.10? Why?

40. Does increasing the alpha increase or decrease the risk of a type one error?

ANSWERS TO ODD-NUMBERED CHAPTER 6 REVIEW QUESTIONS

1. H_0: There is no relationship between years worked and salary earned.

   H_1: There is a relationship between years worked and salary earned. (Or you could write: More years worked is related to a higher earned salary.)

3. Reject the null. The p-value is significant; therefore, you conclude that there is a relationship between years worked and salary earned.

5. You do not know. It depends on the clinical judgment of the experts in clinical care. You may be one of them!

7. Alpha of 0.01

9. Reject the null. There is an association between a positive toxicology screen for Rohypnol and signs of sexual assault.

11. Qualitative

13. $15 \div 45 = 33.3\%$

15. $35 \div 45 = 77.7\%$

17. There is a relationship between the strain of HPV infection and cervical cell abnormalities.

19. Nominal

21. Two-staged cluster sample

23. $62 \div 120 = 52\%$

25. $104 \div 120 = 87\%$

27. CIN I

29. Low-risk

31. Fail to reject the null; $p >$ alpha

33. Reject the null; $p <$ alpha

35. No, in addition to being statistically significant, experts in the field must also support the argument that it is a clinically significant difference.

37.

Study	p-Value	Alpha = 0.05	Alpha = 0.10
A	0.0647	Fail to reject the null	Reject the null
B	0.912	Fail to reject the null	Fail to reject the null
C	0.1567	Fail to reject the null	Fail to reject the null
D	0.0211	Reject the null	Reject the null
E	0.081	Fail to reject the null	Reject the null

39. A, D, E—in order to make a type one error you must reject the null incorrectly.

CHAPTER 7

SAMPLE SIZE, EFFECT SIZE, AND POWER

SO HOW MANY SUBJECTS DO I NEED?

OBJECTIVES

By the end of the chapter students will be able to:

- Describe the components of sample size calculation and relate them to one another.

- Recognize a type two error and contrast it with a type one error.

- Estimate the chance of a type two or type one error in a current research article.

- Interpret the power in a current research study and how it would affect the necessary sample size if it were increased or decreased.

- Calculate the anticipated effect size in a study.

KEY TERMS

Alpha (α)
The chance of making a type one error.

Beta (β)
The chance of making a type two error.

Effect size
The extent to which a difference or relationship exists between variables in a population (the size of the difference you are attempting to find).

Power
The ability to find a difference or an association when one actually exists.

Power analysis
How sample sizes are calculated.

Type one error
The error made when a researcher incorrectly rejects the null hypothesis, when he or she concludes there is a significant relationship but there really is not.

Type two error
The error made when a researcher accepts the null incorrectly, missing an association that is really there (sometimes called a power error because the researcher may not have enough power to find an association that really exists).

EFFECT SIZE

You've gotten pretty far in your research. You've noticed clinical associations, examined descriptive data, evaluated the measurement tools, generated a hypothesis, and decided on your sampling method. Now you need to determine how many subjects you will actually need to sample. This decision is largely dependent on the **effect size**, or the size of the difference between group means that exists within the population.

Effect size and sample size are inversely proportional: As one increases, the other decreases. This fact surprises a lot of people, but it is not too difficult to grasp if you think about it. If you are anticipating a large difference (i.e., a strong effect), you may need only a small sample to detect it. If you are anticipating a small difference (i.e., a weak effect), you may need to collect a very large sample to detect it. For example, if the average weight of adult men in the population is 195 pounds and the average weight of adult women is 166 pounds, there is an almost 30-pound difference in the mean weights in the two samples. You probably wouldn't need a large sample of men and women to show that there is a statistically significant difference in the average weight of adult men and women because there is a large difference in the population means. However, if the average weight of a 35-week fetus is 5.25 pounds and the average weight of a 36-week fetus is 5.78, you would need a larger sample to show a statistically significant difference in a sample of 35-week fetuses and a sample of 36-week fetuses. The closer the two sample means are to each other in the population, the more information you need to demonstrate they are actually different in the sample in your study.

One way to determine effect size mathematically is to divide the difference between the mean in the experimental group and the mean in the control group by the standard deviation of the control group. Some statisticians prefer to delineate small, medium, and large effect sizes based on the statistical procedure being conducted, whereas others use general guidelines such as those that follow.

Let's look at an example. Grove (2007) prefers to use the following values:

- A weak effect size $<$ is 0.3 (or –0.3).
- A moderate effect size is 0.3–0.5 (or 0.3 to 0.5).
- A strong effect size is $>$ 0.5 (or –0.5).

If you want to know how much of an actual difference in means this is, you can multiply the effect size by the standard deviation in the control group. For example, in a study on the effect of an intervention with premature infants, the control group had a standard deviation of 10 days.

- An intervention with a weak effect size would be associated with a decrease of less than 3 days of prematurity (0.1 or 0.2 × 10).
- A moderate effect size would be associated with a decrease of 3–5 days in prematurity (0.3 to 0.5 × 10).

- A decrease in more than 5 days of prematurity would be a large effect size (0.6 [or more] × 10).

Most of the time, the actual effect size in the population is unknown and must be estimated based on the best literature available. Over- or underestimating the effect size can have an impact on the size of the sample collected and the likelihood of reaching an accurate conclusion.

The size of the sample relates directly to the **power** of the study, or the ability to find a difference when one actually exists. The two concepts are directly proportional; that is, as one increases, the other must as well. Thus, when sample size is increased, the power of the study is increased, and the likelihood of rejecting the null hypothesis correctly is increased. Power is defined as the likelihood of rejecting the null hypothesis correctly; that is, you say there is a relationship and difference, and you are correct. It is usually considered adequate to have a power of 0.80, or 80% (Munro, 2005).

FROM THE STATISTICIAN *Brendan Heavey*

The Four Pillars of Study Planning

Whenever I plan a study, particularly in deciding on sample size, I like to think of myself as juggling four mysterious balls that represent each of the following:

- Alpha level
- Effect size
- Power
- Sample size

(continues)

FROM THE STATISTICIAN *Brendan Heavey*

None of these balls is labeled, but knowing any three enables me to know the fourth without seeing any labels.

The **alpha** level is the probability of rejecting H_0 (the null hypothesis) given that it is true. For our present purposes, setting alpha to 0.05 every time is acceptable.

Think of *effect size* as the amount of difference between what was hypothesized in H_0 and what we find in our study. When planning a study, we try to ensure that true differences result in statistical significance, but false differences do not. So the smaller the difference is that we want to detect, the larger the number of cases we need to look at. (Effect size is inversely proportional to sample size.)

How does the researcher decide on the size of the difference to look at? This is not a statistical question; it has to be determined by previous studies or by some other scientific means. This determination can be tricky. Statisticians rely heavily on investigators to provide them with a difference that is clinically important. Determining the degree of difference can be a major undertaking and requires much background research. Sometimes figuring this out takes longer than completing the whole study!

The third concept, power, is probably the most difficult concept to grasp in any introductory statistics class. Many beginning students have trouble understanding it. You can think of power as the probability of rejecting the null hypothesis when the alternative hypothesis is true. Power depends on the truth of the hypothesis under study and totally ignores what happens when the null hypothesis is true. Other analysis methods (specifically, setting an alpha threshold) take into account when the null hypothesis is true. Power takes the analysis a step further.

Most studies typically consider 80% power as adequate; that is, if the alternative hypothesis is true, you have a probability of at least 80% that you will reject the null hypothesis. This standard percentage is based on convention, just like having an alpha of 0.05. To increase power (the probability of rejecting the null when the alternative is true) and maintain the same alpha level (the probability of incorrectly rejecting the null), you need to increase the sample size. In simpler terms, increasing power requires increasing sample size in order to maintain the same alpha level. Power is *directly* proportional to sample size: When sample size increases, power increases. If you want to increase power, increase your sample size.

Sample size (represented as *n*) is the fourth ball juggled in study planning. Statisticians *always* want to increase sample size. Increasing sample size is rarely a bad thing. The problem is that increasing sample size usually means increasing the cost of a study, so statisticians use other approaches to decide on an acceptable sample size.

There are two usual ways of planning a study. The first involves defining the desired effect size and then figuring out the sample size needed to achieve the related power. Statisticians usually choose 0.80, or 80%, power and then decide whether the study is possible given the required sample size. In other words, the juggler in me:

- Selects alpha (juggled object 1) as 0.05.
- Defines the effect size of interest (juggled object 2).
- Sets power to 80% (juggled object 3).
- This leaves me with one last juggling object, the sample size, which is completely determined by the other three. The equations you will use to make these determinations are determined by the statistical technique you will employ in your study.

I then do a cost/benefit analysis on my final sample size to determine whether the study should be done. For example, if the cost of acquiring the necessary data for an adequately sized sample is $100,000, I have to determine whether the benefit associated with the anticipated results will have a value greater than this investment.

Another approach to study planning is to determine what sample size is available and then what effect size is needed to achieve the appropriate power level (again, usually 0.80, or 80%). In this case, alpha is again set to 0.05; sample size is set to our determined limit; and power is set to 0.80, or 80%. That leaves the juggled object of effect size to be figured out, and it can now be determined based on the other three. Finally, the researcher must determine whether the effect size is interesting enough to warrant performing the study (this usually involves a cost/benefit analysis).

For instance, oversupplementation of vitamin A has been shown to cause liver damage. We design a study to determine whether the damage is caused by reduced blood flow to the liver. We have been given a National Institutes of Health award for outstanding merit in clinical research based on our previous work with EpiPens. The award is for $500,000 and must be put toward further research. With this amount, we can enroll 25 subjects in our study ($n = 25$), who will be asked to come to the hospital for 4 hours, fill out a survey, have blood drawn, and undergo a positron emission tomography (PET) scan. We set the alpha level at 0.05 and power at 0.8, or 80%, which we figure will be sufficient to predict an increase of 0.8 mL/min/g of blood flow or higher. Unfortunately, with this size sample, we can detect only a very large difference (i.e., effect size) in blood flow to the liver. By the time patients have that much difference in blood flow to the liver, they will have already exhibited other detectable signs and symptoms of liver disease, so the effect size we could find with this sample size is too large to be clinically useful. We need to be able to find a smaller difference for the results to be clinically useful; specifically, the study would be useful only if we can predict a difference of 0.08 mL/min/g or lower. Detecting this small an effect size requires us to enroll more subjects than we can afford with this grant money.

Can you figure out what other factors we might adjust to make this study feasible? That's the juggling act.

These four concepts are all interrelated. Changing one can affect all three of the others. Note that alpha is rarely changed to accommodate lack of funding. Instead, we first reduce power because, in the scientific community, it is generally worse to give up on answers that might be right than it is to waste time on answers that are probably wrong. We'll look at this reasoning in more depth in the next "From the Statistician."

TYPE TWO ERROR

Anytime you make a decision, there is a chance that you will make a mistake (like ordering garlic sushi on a blind date—big mistake!). When your decision involves failing to reject the null hypothesis, you must consider the possibility of a **type two error**, that is, the error made when you fail to reject the null *incorrectly*, thus missing an association that is really there. These errors usually occur because the sample wasn't large enough and the study therefore didn't have enough power to find a difference that really existed. Hence type two errors are also frequently called power errors.

Any hypothesis test has the risk of committing a type two error. This risk is represented by **beta (β)**. You can calculate your chance of a type two error fairly simply. Given that there really is a relationship or difference between the variables you are examining, you will either correctly identify it (i.e., reject H_0 correctly = power) or you will incorrectly miss it (type two error). Because there is a 100% chance that you will be *either* correct *or* incorrect (pretty much true for all life decisions), you know that:

Power (correctly rejecting H_0) + Beta (chance of making a type two error) = 100%

Therefore, if there is an 80% chance that you are correct and find the relationship (power), the chance of a type two error is 20%.

On a practical basis, the convention is to set beta at 20%. You can quickly calculate beta by subtracting the power of the study (usually 80%, or 0.80) from one: $1 - 0.80 = 0.20$.

A QUICK REVIEW OF TYPE ONE AND TYPE TWO ERRORS

Type one and type two errors seem relatively straightforward until you start trying to think about both of them together. Sort them out like this. The life decisions rule is that, no matter what you are deciding, there are usually two outcomes: You are (1) correct or (2) incorrect. (All of the philosopher-students are horrified that I see things this way, but bear with me.) The question that all research studies ask is whether the null hypothesis is true: The two variables have no relationship, difference, or association between them. In actuality, it may be true or it may not be true, and you can reject or fail to reject the null hypothesis in either of these situations.

If the null hypothesis really *is* true and there is no relationship or difference between the variables, you can conclude one of two things:

- You can fail to reject it. You are *correct* in this situation, and the probability of reaching this conclusion is $1 - \alpha$ (usually 0.05), or 95%.
- Or you can reject it. Then you are incorrect and are making a **type one error**. The probability of reaching this conclusion is equal to α, usually 5%.

If the null hypothesis is really not true and there is a relationship between the variables, you can conclude one of two things:

- You can fail to reject it. In this case, you are *incorrect* and are making a type two error. The probability of doing so is equal to β (usually 0.20, or 20%).
- You can reject it *correctly*. The probability of reaching this conclusion is $1 - \beta$ (usually 80%), which is also the power of your study.

Getting the two types of errors confused is easy, so thinking of them in terms of the null hypothesis is helpful. If you reject the null *and are incorrect*, you are making a type one error. If you fail to reject the null *and are incorrect*, you are making a type two error (see **Figure 7-1**). Of course, if you are already a statistician, you

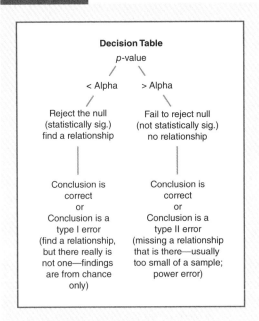

FIGURE 7-1   **Thinking It Through.**

may not need this tip—but the rest of us get confused sometimes!

SAMPLE SIZE

All these ideas are related, and you need to understand them to determine your sample size. Before you even begin a study, you need to decide how many subjects to sample. That decision depends on the size of the difference you are looking to detect. In other words, the sample size you need should give you adequate power to reject the null hypothesis correctly. **Power analysis** is how sample sizes are calculated. The many different equations for calculating sample sizes depend on the statistical techniques the study utilizes. Luckily for you, these calculations are beyond the scope of this text. (So you have something to look forward to in your next stats class!) However, power analysis involves some central concepts no matter which calculation you are using. The sample size you need in your study depends on the following:

- *Effect size:* The anticipated difference you expect to see
- *How much type one error you can tolerate:* Alpha, or chances of incorrectly saying there is a difference
- *Power:* The ability to detect a difference that really exists

Even after calculating the necessary sample size, you may need to increase it if you anticipate a large number of dropouts or a high nonresponse rate. For example, many nurses who are asked about their sexual orientation may choose not to respond to that question, leaving you with too small a sample size to draw any conclusions. If you are conducting a study over a long period of time, a number of participants will be lost to follow-up or will

FROM THE STATISTICIAN *Brendan Heavey*

Which Error Is Worse? The Lesser of Two Evils

How do we decide how many subjects to enroll for a study? This is a bread-and-butter question for statisticians, and their answer involves a concept that many people don't understand. Often statisticians have to decide whether it is worse to commit a type one error or a type two error. Statisticians can debate the question for hours, but in this country's legal system—as well as in most of the world's scientific community and real-life situations—committing a type one error is definitely worse.

Let me explain that point. In any court case, four different scenarios are possible, just as in the hypothesis test explanation (see **Table 7-1**). The U.S. legal system is based on the principle that people are innocent until proven guilty (H_0: The defendant is not guilty). Inherent in that principle is a subprinciple that sending an innocent person to jail is much worse than letting a guilty person walk. This is the reason for such an enormous appeals process and why you cannot be tried twice for the same offense.

(continues)

FROM THE STATISTICIAN *Brendan Heavey*

TABLE 7-1	**Criminal Status and Trial Results**		
		Truth	
		Defendant Is Innocent	**Defendant Is Guilty**
Result of the trial	Defendant is convicted.	Major problem; TYPE ONE ERROR	No problem; $1 - \beta$ = power
	Defendant is acquitted.	No problem; $1 - a$	Minor problem; TYPE TWO ERROR

In statistics we have a similar philosophy:

- We put a hard cap on alpha (the probability of a false positive) of about 0.05.
- We shoot for a power of about 80%.
- So beta, the probability of a false negative, is set around 0.20 (a much more likely outcome than the accepted probability for a false positive).

We do the same thing in statistics that the U.S. court system does; we just charge less per hour than the average lawyer!

Medical researchers play by much the same rules. Often, researchers find sets of genes that they think may be involved in causing cancer or some other debilitating disease. Once they have found a set of interest, the next step is to test all of them simultaneously in groups of control versus cancerous subjects. This research process can involve upward of 50,000 genes in thousands of subjects at once. What would go through your head if you had to decide how to run this large and complex analysis? You would have to sort each gene into one of the four categories from the 2 × 2 table. Most of the genes would have the same expression in both cancerous and control tissue, and you could eliminate them from contention. Beyond that set, you'd have to decide which is worse: rejecting the one lone gene that may be the cause of cancer *or* wasting time sifting through too many genes that don't have anything to do with your analysis question. Obviously, rejecting the right answer is the worse of the two evils. Unfortunately, this means that scientists' time gets wasted all too often!

be unable to participate for various reasons, such as death, illness, relocation, and the like. These factors all need to be considered when calculating the number of subjects to include in a sample.

When a sample size is too small, you have a greater chance of a type two error. If you don't have enough subjects, you may not find a statistical difference even though one exists. However, when the sample is too large, you not only waste time and money but also have a greater chance of a type one error. You might find a statistical difference that really isn't there and promote a treatment or course of action that may not be the best option for patients.

All of this information about sample size applies to quantitative studies; however, you will see that some qualitative studies have much smaller samples and utilize a technique called sampling to saturation. This simply means collecting subject interviews until the researchers determine the interviews are not producing any additional new data or themes. Qualitative studies utilize very different analysis techniques; thus, smaller samples may still yield promising results.

SUMMARY

Way to go! You have completed the chapter. Now for a quick review.

- The effect size is the extent to which a difference or relationship exists between the variables under study in the population. It is also the size or difference you are attempting to find in your study.
- The power of the study is the ability to find a difference when one actually does exist.
- A power analysis is how sample sizes are actually calculated.
- A type one error is rejecting the null hypothesis incorrectly. In other words, the researcher states that there is a difference in the variables when there really isn't one.
- A type two error is failing to reject the null incorrectly, meaning that the researcher misses a relationship that does exist.
- Beta is another name for the chance of committing a type two error.
- The sample size you need in your study depends on the effect size or the anticipated difference you expect to see.

CHAPTER 7 REVIEW QUESTIONS

Questions 1–14: You are asked to develop a study for a pharmaceutical company to determine whether taking one tablet of drug A is related to lower total cholesterol levels.

1. What is your independent variable?

2. What is your dependent variable?

3. How could you measure your dependent variable quantitatively?

   A. Would this be a continuous or categorical variable?

   B. What level of measurement would this variable be?

4. How could you measure your dependent variable qualitatively?

   A. Would this be a continuous or categorical variable?

   B. What level of measurement would this variable be?

5. You chose to measure taking one tablet of drug A as a yes-or-no question.

   A. What level of measurement is this variable?

   B. What would be the best measure of central tendency?

6. Write a null hypothesis for your study.

7. Write an alternative hypothesis for your study.

8. If you select an alpha of 0.05 and a power of 80%, what does your decision mean?

9. Your study has an alpha of 0.05. Your statistical test determines that the p-value for the relationship between taking one tablet of drug A daily and lowering cholesterol is 0.02. What do you conclude?

10. If your conclusion was actually a type one error, what do you know about taking drug A and cholesterol levels?

11. Based on the preliminary pilot study you conducted, the drug company decides to fund a large-scale clinical trial. This trial results in a *p*-value of 0.07. What is your conclusion?

12. You determine after the trial that the actual effect size from the medication was smaller than you initially thought. Your conclusion may be what type of error?

13. What was the most likely cause of this error?

14. If your study had an alpha of 0.05 and a power of 80%, calculate the chance that you made a type two error.

15. In each of the following instances, identify which type of error is potentially being made: type one or type two.

    A. Your study concludes that ambulation post-op day 1 from hip replacement surgery is associated with shorter hospital stays.

    B. Your study examining the relationship between head trauma and grand mal seizures has an alpha of 0.10 and a beta of 0.80. Your statistical analysis reports a *p*-value of 0.06.

    C. Your study finds no relationship between vitamin E consumption and skin cancer.

    D. Your original intention was to enroll 500 subjects in your study, but only 256 completed both a pre- and posttest. You are concerned about what type of error?

    E. Your study has an alpha of 0.05 and a beta of 0.90. You examine a sample of circus workers to determine whether they have higher levels of lung cancer. Your statistical analysis finds a *p*-value of 0.04.

    F. The poorly designed pilot study examining the relationship between mold exposure and asthma reports a small effect size. You recruit a large sample to attempt to enable your research team to detect this effect size successfully. Having a larger sample size increases the risk of making what type of error?

16. You have two samples of adults preparing for barium enema tests the next day. The control group consumes 2 oz of milk of magnesia with a mean average of 120 ml and a standard deviation of 10 ml of water. The second group is advised to consume more water with their milk of magnesia, and they average 124 ml with a standard deviation of 12 ml of water. Calculate the effect size in this experiment. Is it small, moderate, or large by Grove's standards?

Questions 17–30: A study anticipates that subjects treated with drug A will have substantial improvement in their neuropathy symptoms.

17. If the study measures treatment with drug A as given or not given, what level of measurement is this variable?

18. If the study measures treatment with drug A as not given, low dose, or high dose, what level of measurement is this variable?

19. If the study measures treatment with drug A as 0 mg/day, 100 mg/day, or 200 mg/day, what level of measurement is this variable?

20. If the study measures neuropathy symptoms as present or not present, what level of measurement is this variable?

21. If the study measures neuropathy symptoms on a scale of 1–10, what level of measurement is this variable?

22. If the study measures neuropathy symptoms as mild, moderate, or severe, what level of measurement is this variable?

23. The study anticipates subjects treated with drug A will have substantial improvement in their neuropathy symptoms. What effect size is anticipated, and what does that mean in terms of the sample size needed?

24. The researcher knows of a validated survey instrument to measure neuropathy symptoms, but it has 500 questions and requires a college-level reading ability to understand. These features limit what aspect of the measurement tool?

25. The 10-question survey instrument used to measure neuropathy symptoms in this study was compared to a previously validated 500-question version, and similar results were obtained. This is an example of establishing what type of validity?

26. This large-scale trial will have measurements collected by 14 data collectors at three sites. Discuss an aspect of reliability that will be critical to assess and thus avoid compromising the validity of the study.

27. The neuropathy survey has a 96% sensitivity. What does this mean?

28. This study, which examines treating patients with drug A and neuropathy symptoms, utilizes an alpha of 0.05 and reports a *p*-value of 0.30. What should the researcher decide about the null hypothesis? Why?

29. If this decision in review question 28 about the null hypothesis is incorrect, what type of error could it be?

30. In the following table, fill in the researcher's decision about the null hypothesis at the indicated alpha level as well as what potential error it could be if this decision is incorrect.

p-Value	Alpha Value	Null Hypothesis Decision	Potential Error
0.061	0.05		
0.101	0.05		
0.022	0.05		
0.167	0.10		
0.014	0.10		
0.079	0.05		
0.079	0.10		

31. If a researcher reports that the abuse of dextromethorphan is not related to age but is incorrect about this conclusion, what type of error is this?

32. A researcher reports that exposure to fentanyl patches is associated with death in children. What does this mean about the relationship between the *p*-value and the alpha in the study? If this conclusion is an error, what type would it be?

33. A researcher reports a statistically significant association between taking anticoagulants and bruising. What do you know about the sample size?

34. The researchers are trying to detect a small effect size. What do you know about the necessary sample size?

35. Researchers report that there is no difference in appetite for those taking Byetta and those who are not. However, the sample size was small, and the results are incorrect. This is what type of error?

ANSWERS TO ODD-NUMBERED CHAPTER 7 REVIEW QUESTIONS

1. Drug A

3. Serum cholesterol, (a) continuous, (b) interval/ratio

5. (a) nominal, (b) mode

7. Answers may vary. Examples: (1) Taking drug A is associated with a change in cholesterol level. (2) Drug A lowers cholesterol level.

9. Reject the null hypothesis. There is a relationship between taking drug A and cholesterol levels.

11. Fail to reject the null; there is not enough evidence to show a relationship between drug A and cholesterol levels.

13. Inadequate power due to too small of a sample to detect this effect size

15. a. Reject the null; may be a type one error.
    b. Reject the null; may be a type one error.
    c. Fail to reject the null; may be a type two error.
    d. Fail to reject the null; may be a type two error due to inadequate sample.

e. Reject the null; may be a type one error.
f. Reject the null; may be a type one error.

17. Nominal

19. Ratio

21. Interval

23. Large effect size is anticipated, so only a small sample should be necessary to detect it on a statistically significant level.

25. Convergent validity

27. If the patient has neuropathy, there is a 96% chance that the survey will indicate this result.

29. Type two

31. Type two

33. It was adequate to detect the effect size.

35. Type two

CHAPTER 8

CHI-SQUARE

IS THERE A DIFFERENCE?

OBJECTIVES

By the end of the chapter students will be able to:

- Identify conditions under which the chi-square test is appropriate.
- Identify the question that the chi-square test is designed to answer.
- Formulate a null and an alternative hypothesis.
- Formulate a 2 × 2 table from an existing data set.
- Interpret a Statistical Package for the Social Sciences (SPSS) printout of a chi-square test, determine what action to take with regard to the null hypothesis,

and justify this decision in statistically correct terminology.

- Identify a current research article that uses a chi-square test, determine the level of measurement of the variables used and whether the results are statistically significant, and utilize this information to draw a statistical conclusion.
- Debate whether clinical recommendations should be made from a research article's conclusion, and prepare a public health report using this information.

KEY TERMS

Chi-square (X^2)
A test used with independent samples of nominal- or ordinal-level data.

Degrees of freedom (df)
The number values that are "free to be unknown."

Null hypothesis
No relationship, association, or difference exists between the variables of interest.

CHI-SQUARE (X^2) TEST

Recall that, in most experiments, the **null hypothesis** means that no relationship, association, or difference exists between the study groups or samples. So how can we test to see whether there really is no difference? That's what we will discuss here: an actual test to see whether there is a statistically significant difference.

In this chapter, we are going to talk about the **chi-square (X^2)** test, which is appropriate when you are working with independent samples and an outcome or dependent variable that is nominal- or ordinal-level data. You already know that nominal-level data tells you that there is a difference in the quality of a variable, whereas ordinal-level data has a rank-order so that one level is greater than or less than another.

For example, suppose you are an operating room nurse, and you want to see whether there is a difference between male and female postoperative patients in the need for a postoperative transfusion. Gender is the variable that identifies your sample groups. You want to compare a sample of men and a sample of women. Your outcome or dependent variable is postoperative transfusion, which is measured at a nominal level (yes or no). Now you want to see whether the frequencies you observe are different from the frequencies you would expect if the variables were independent, or not related.

THE NULL AND ALTERNATIVE HYPOTHESES

Let's formulate a null hypothesis and an alternative hypothesis using the standard notation, which looks like this:

H_0: This is how statisticians indicate the null hypothesis.
H_1: This notation indicates the alternative hypothesis.

Here are our hypotheses:

H_0: There is no difference in the need for a postoperative transfusion among men and women.
H_1: The need for a postoperative transfusion is different for men and women.

2×2 TABLE

Your next step is to set up another 2×2 table. Statisticians love these! See **Table 8-1**.

TABLE 8-1	**Gender and Postoperative Transfusion Status**		
	Male	**Female**	**Total**
Transfused	20 (A)	40 (B)	60 (A + B)
Not Transfused	30 (C)	10 (D)	40 (C + D)
Total	50 (A + C)	50 (B + D)	100 (A + B + C + D)

DEGREES OF FREEDOM

Before you determine statistical significance, you need to determine the **degrees of freedom (*df*)**, which is the number values that are "free to be unknown" once the row and column totals are in a 2 × 2 contingency table. With a chi-square test, the degrees of freedom are equal to the number of rows minus one times the number of columns minus one:

$$df = (2-1) \times (2-1)$$
$$df = 1 \times 1 = 1$$

All 2 × 2 tables have one degree of freedom. In other words, once you know the row and column totals and one other cell value in the table, you can figure out the rest of the cell values in the table, and they do not change unless the original cell value changes. This is why there is only one value that is "free to be unknown."

STATISTICAL SIGNIFICANCE

Once you put your data into a statistical program, it will compute the expected values for each of these cells, assuming that the two variables are independent. You will then need to apply the chi-square test to see whether the observed values are significantly different from the expected values at one degree of freedom.

- If the X^2 result has a *p*-value that is significant (usually 0.05, depending on the alpha you use), then you reject the null hypothesis that the two variables are independent and conclude that there is an association between gender and postoperative transfusion. Postoperative transfusion rates are significantly different for men and women.
- If the X^2 result has a *p*-value that is greater than the alpha you selected (e.g., if your alpha is 0.05 and the *p*-value is 0.09), then the result is not statistically significant and you fail to reject the null hypothesis. Your study does not have the statistical strength for you to say that the variables are not related. In this case you conclude that postoperative transfusion rates are not significantly different for men and women. Remember that this may be because there really isn't a difference in postoperative transfusion rates for men and women or because of another reason, such as your sample size was too small.

DIRECTION OF THE RELATIONSHIP

Also note that the chi-square test doesn't tell you the direction of the relationship or difference. If the *p*-value for your X^2 is significant, all you know is that you can reject the null and that there is a statistically significant difference in your outcome variable between the two samples. As the statistical wizard that you are, you then look again at your data to determine that difference. For example, if you had a statistically significant X^2 in the example about gender and postoperative transfusions, you could go back and look at which gender had more transfusions. In this sample, a larger portion of the women needed transfusions. Given your statistically significant result, you could conclude that, for this sample, women are more likely to need a postoperative transfusion than men.

FROM THE STATISTICIAN *Brendan Heavey*

Pearson's Chi-Square Test for Association

The chi-square test is one of the simplest tests available in a subset of statistics called categorical data analysis. The majority of theories relating to categorical data analysis started to be developed around the turn of the 20th century. Karl Pearson (1857–1936) was a very important statistician from England who is responsible for first developing the chi-squared distribution. Pearson was an arrogant man who frequently butted heads with colleagues. He specifically argued the intelligence and merits of a young statistician named R. A. Fisher (1890–1962), who has since become established as one of the most important scientists of all time. The two men argued over many different things. Fisher was concerned about what would happen to Pearson's chi-squared statistic when sample sizes were extremely low, and Pearson didn't think it was a problem.

Fisher contributed a number of fundamentals of statistical science, and he developed the Fisher exact test. This test is now commonly used in place of Pearson's chi-square test when the sample size of any cell in the data is less than 5 (because, in the end, Fisher's arguments with Pearson proved correct). Fisher also used properties derived from Pearson's chi-squared distribution to show that Gregor Mendel, the eminent geneticist and Augustinian priest who theorized about the inheritance of genetic traits using peas, most likely derived many of his theories based on fabricated data. (Fisher remained convinced that one of Mendel's assistants was responsible for the fabrication; Mendel is still considered a very gifted geneticist.) In any event, the two tests—Pearson's chi-square test and Fisher's exact test—are now very common statistics to use in clinical trials and scientific research. Specifically, their use is very popular when a researcher wants to test whether a new treatment or therapy is better than the so-called gold standard already in use.

The null hypothesis that is tested in both these tests is:

H_0: The proportions being compared are equal in the population.

Here is a motivating example, one that's slightly more difficult than the one in the main text. This time we'll use a variable that has more than just two categories.

Suppose we want to study the effect of a husband's occupation on a woman's marital happiness in a clinically relevant population. Our null hypothesis is:

H_0: Husband's occupation has no effect on women's marital happiness in this subset of occupations in the population we have sampled from.

FROM THE STATISTICIAN *Brendan Heavey*

To conduct the study, we enroll 1,868 women and ask them to rate the happiness of their marriage on the following four-point scale:

- Very happy
- Pretty happy
- Happy
- Not too happy

The results are shown in **Table 8-2**. Now, if you plug these values into any statistical program (or use the From the Statistician: Methods section from this chapter to hand-calculate the values), you'll see that the *p*-value for the difference between the happiness of the wives of statisticians versus those of male supermodels is so low that it is estimated at 0. Now you know that there is an association between the husband's occupation and the wife's marital happiness (because your *p*-value is less than alpha, meaning it is significant). So you reject the null hypothesis that there isn't a relationship between a husband's occupation and a wife's marital happiness.

But what else might you like to know? Let's say that a friend is dating a statistician and a male supermodel and that they both intend to propose this evening. What advice would you give your friend? Which might be the better choice to ensure long-term marital satisfaction? Remember that the chi-square test tells you only that there is a better choice, not which one it is. But you remember from your college stats class that you can determine which is better by looking at the data. The proportion of wives married to statisticians who reported being happy or higher was 99.9% (1,706 ÷ 1,708), whereas the proportion of wives married to supermodels who reported being happy or higher was 37.5% (60 ÷ 160). Assuming that your friend wants to get married in the first place, which proposal should she accept? (*Hint:* In the statistics books, the statisticians always live happily ever after!)

| TABLE 8-2 | **Husbands' Occupation and Wives' Report of Marital Happiness** |

	Husbands' Occupation		
Marital Happiness	**Statistician**	**Male Supermodel**	**Total**
Very happy	800	25	825
Pretty happy	706	10	716
Happy	200	25	225
Not too happy	2	100	102
Total	1,708	160	1,868

(continues)

FROM THE STATISTICIAN *Brendan Heavey*

Here are three health-related studies that all demonstrate the use of this statistic:

- Corless et al. (2009) examined the effect of marijuana use versus over-the-counter medications for the relief of symptoms and side effects associated with HIV medication.
- Tobian et al. (2009) investigated the contribution of different variables to determine whether circumcision was an effective strategy for syphilis prevention in a community in Uganda.
- Anifantaki (2009) examined the relationship between daily interruption of sedative infusions and the duration of mechanical ventilation required in patients in an adult surgical intensive care unit.

Note: All the anecdotal information regarding Spearman and Fisher came from Agresti's (2002) landmark book on the subject, *Categorical Data Analysis*.

WHEN NOT TO USE CHI-SQUARE: ASSUMPTIONS AND SPECIAL CASES

In a few situations, you might be inclined to use a chi-square test because you have an outcome or dependent variable at the nominal level, but the test wouldn't be a good choice. The chi-square test includes some additional assumptions (in addition to requiring a nominal-level outcome or dependent variable), which must be met for the test to be used appropriately.

All cells within the 2 × 2 table must have an expected value greater than or equal to 5. If at least one cell in your 2 × 2 table has an expected value less than 5, you should use the Fisher exact test instead. You should also note that *if any of the cells in the frequency table has greater than 5 but fewer than 10 expected observations*, you can still use the chi-square test, but you need to do a Yates continuity correction as well. The really nice thing in this day and age is that many statistical programs automatically make this

correction when this condition occurs, saving you the time and trouble of doing it manually. You might want to look for it on your next SPSS printout.

The sample should be random and independent. Here's an example of a violation of this assumption: Your study involved measuring the need for postoperative transfusion among husbands and wives who underwent a particular procedure. (Because these subjects are related to each other, they are not independent—once you included the wife in the study, the husband was included as well, so his participation was "dependent" on his wife being selected to participate.) In this case, the sample is not independent and random. Instead, the sample is now matched, or paired, and a test called the McNemar test is the correct choice to use for the analysis. (Both the Fisher and the McNemar tests are based on the same idea as the chi-square, but they have mathematical adjustments to accommodate the violation of the assumptions of the chi-square test.)

THINKING IT THROUGH

Looking for a Difference in Two Samples When the Outcome Variable Is Nominal or Ordinal

Sample Type	Level of Dependent or Outcome Variable	Test	Research Example
Two **independent** samples	**Nominal or ordinal**	Chi-square	Is there a difference in the level of nursing education achieved for male and female nurses? (Independent variable is nominal, male/female, dependent variable is ordinal with four levels: ADN, BSN, MS, and DNP.)
Two **dependent** samples	**Nominal or ordinal**	McNemar's test	In motor vehicle accidents involving a passenger and a driver, is the driver or the passenger more likely to experience a head injury? (Independent variables of driver and passenger are related because they are in the same car and therefore create two dependent samples; the dependent variable head injury is yes or no, or nominal.)

Note: Samples or groups can be created by the levels of the independent variable. For example, gender may be your independent variable, and the groups you are interested in comparing are men and women, creating two samples or groups to compare.)

FROM THE STATISTICIAN *Brendan Heavey*

Methods: Calculating Pearson's Chi-Square Test by Hand

Table 8-3 is a repeat of Table 8-2, for easier reference.

- The first step is to calculate the expected frequency from each cell with the following formula:

$$\text{Expected frequency} = \frac{\text{Row total} \times \text{Column total}}{\text{Grand total}}$$

The results are shown in **Table 8-4**.

- Now compute the statistic:

$$\sum \frac{\left(\text{Observed} - \text{Expected}\right)^2}{\text{Expected}}$$

(continues)

FROM THE STATISTICIAN *Brendan Heavey*

TABLE 8-3   Husbands' Occupation and Wives' Report of Marital Happiness

Marital Happiness	Husbands' Occupation		
	Statistician	Male Supermodel	Total
Very happy	800	25	825
Pretty happy	706	10	716
Happy	200	25	225
Not too happy	2	100	102
Total	1,708	160	1,868

TABLE 8-4   Expected Frequencies for Husbands' Occupation and Wives' Marital Satisfaction

	Expected Frequencies	
	Statistician	Male Supermodel
Very happy	$(825 \times 1{,}708) \div 1868 = 754.34$	$(825 \times 160) \div 1{,}868 = 70.66$
Pretty happy	$(716 \times 1{,}708) \div 1868 = 654.67$	$(716 \times 160) \div 1{,}868 = 61.33$
Happy	$(225 \times 1{,}708) \div 1868 = 205.73$	$(225 \times 160) \div 1{,}868 = 19.27$
Not too happy	$(102 \times 1{,}708) \div 1868 = 93.26$	$(102 \times 160) \div 1{,}868 = 8.74$

The big sigma character (Σ) just means to sum everything over all the cells; in our case we calculate:

$$\frac{(800-754.34)^2}{754.37} + \frac{(706-654.67)^2}{654.67} + \frac{(200-205.73)^2}{205.73} + \frac{(2-93.26)^2}{93.26}$$

$$+ \frac{(25-70.66)^2}{70.66} + \frac{(10-61.33)^2}{61.33} + \frac{(200-205.73)^2}{19.27} + \frac{(2-93.26)^2}{8.74}$$

which results in 1123.8.

FROM THE STATISTICIAN *Brendan Heavey*

- We then apply the formula for calculating the degrees of freedom for a chi-square test:

$$(\text{Number of rows} - 1)(\text{Number of columns} - 1)$$

  In this case, the degrees of freedom are:

$$3 \times 1 = 3$$

- We can then look up the *p*-value for this test statistic from a table of the chi-square distribution with degrees of freedom:

$$p < 0.0001.$$

SUMMARY

There are two main points to review in this chapter. First, you should understand the concept of the null hypothesis. The null hypothesis means that no relationship, association, or difference exists between the variables of interest. Second, the chi-square test is used to look for a statistically significant difference or relationship when you have a nominal- or ordinal-level dependent or outcome variable.

- If the chi-square test result has a *p*-value that is significant (less than 0.05 or whatever alpha you use), then you reject the null hypothesis.
- If the chi-square test result is not statistically significant (greater than 0.05 or the alpha of choice), then you fail to reject the null hypothesis.

Don't forget to use your decision tree! See **Figure 8-1**.

Last, the chi-square test does not tell you the direction of the relationship; only you can make that interpretation.

That wraps up this chapter. Not too bad, right?

FIGURE 8-1   **Thinking It Through.**

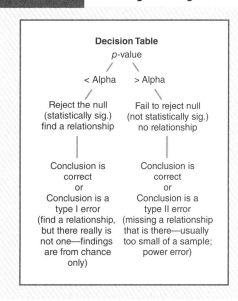

CHAPTER 8 REVIEW QUESTIONS

Questions 1–11: A study is completed to examine the relationship between gender and sports participation. It is conducted by randomly surveying ninth-graders at Smith High School. The collected data is shown in **Table 8-5**.

TABLE 8-5	**Gender and Sports Participation among Ninth-Grade Students**		
	Male	**Female**	**Total**
No sports	30	50	80
Sports participation	70	50	120
Total	100	100	200

1. What level of measurement is gender? Is it continuous or categorical?

2. What level of measurement is sports participation? Is it qualitative or quantitative?

3. What measure of central tendency can you determine for sports participation? What is the measure of central tendency for males only? Is the measure of central tendency different for the whole sample?

4. If the whole school has 800 students and the ninth grade has 250 students, what percentage of the ninth-grade population did you sample?

5. Write an appropriate null hypothesis for this study.

6. Write two alternative hypotheses that correspond to your null hypothesis.

7. Calculate the chi-square from the 2 × 2 table in Table 8-5. The *p*-value is < 0.005. Is sports participation significantly different for males and females in this sample? (See the "From the Statistician": Methods calculation.)

8. What should you conclude about your null hypothesis?

9. What type of error might you be making?

10. If you wanted to make the chance of this type of error smaller, what could you do?

11. Why is the chi-square test appropriate for this study?

Questions 12–14: After the school instituted a new aerobics program, data was gathered in a follow-up survey administered in all the grades. The collected information is shown in **Table 8-6**.

12. If the entire school has a population of 800, what percentage of the students are included in your sample?

TABLE 8-6	**Gender and Sports Participation after New Aerobics Program**		
	Male	**Female**	**Total**
No sports	60	20	80
Sports participation	140	180	320
Total	200	200	400

Chi-square = 25, *p* < 0.0001.

13. Is gender related to sports participation in this follow-up survey? If so, which gender is more likely to participate? How many degrees of freedom do you have?

14. Imagine you are the editor of the journal in which an article was submitted for review using a chi-square test to determine whether boys or girls are more likely to participate in sports. After reading it, you realize that the male and female subjects were recruited as brother and sister pairs. What would you conclude about the analysis?

15. You are working in a school-based health center and have developed a new screening tool for suicide risk among adolescent athletes. The pilot of your new screening tool reports that female athletes are more likely to attempt suicide compared with male athletes. These results agree with other published reports from the general adolescent population. This helps establish what type of validity for your new screening tool?

16. You administer your new screening tool in your health clinic but find the results confusing. After reviewing your screening tool, you realize that the following mistake was made: When the survey was administered to three of the male sports teams, it was printed on only one side of the paper and should have been copied onto both sides. As a result, half of the survey was missing when it was administered to these three teams. Is your screen reliable? What does this tell you about the validity of the screening tool in this situation?

17. You correct the copying problem and readminister the screening tool at another school. After 1 year of follow-up, you get the results shown in **Table 8-7**. Explain what each box means in plain English.

TABLE 8-7	**Suicide Risk and Screening Results**		
	Attempted Suicide	**No Suicide Attempt**	**Total**
Screen positive	20	5	25
Screen negative	10	215	225
Total	30	220	250

18. What is the sensitivity of your screen? What does this mean in plain English?

19. What is the specificity of your screen? What does this mean in plain English?

_____

_____

20. What is the positive predictive value (PPV) of your screen? What does this mean in plain English?

_____

_____

21. What is the negative predictive value (NPV) of your screen? What does this mean in plain English?

_____

_____

22. What is the prevalence of suicide attempts in this sample?

_____

_____

23. "From the Statistician" Review Question: Would you do the analysis differently if no women were happily married to male supermodels in the "From the Statistician" feature in this chapter?

_____

_____

Questions 24–33: In a random sample of 100 patients with biopsy-confirmed breast cancer, a study examines cancer detection rates with 50 previously collected, two-dimensional (2D) mammograms compared to detection rates in 50 previously collected, three-dimensional (3D) mammograms. The alpha selected for this pilot study is 0.10, and the power is 0.80.

24. Write a null and an alternative hypothesis for this study.

_____

_____

25. What is the independent variable? What level of measurement is it?

_____

_____

26. What is the dependent variable?

_____

_____

27. If cancer detection is measured as yes or no, what level of measurement is this variable?

28. The pilot study reports a chi-square of 2.46. Is there a significant difference between cancer detection rates with these two screening mechanisms?

29. The study reports 2D mammograms detected 70% of cancers and 3D mammograms detected 90% of cancers with a $p = 0.12$. What decision should the researcher make about the null hypothesis?

30. In a larger study with the same parameters, 2D mammograms detected 75% of cancers and 3D mammograms detected 91% of cancers with a $p = 0.01$. What decision should the researcher make about the null hypothesis?

31. Knowing the results of the larger study should make the researcher wonder if the conclusion of the smaller pilot study was what type of error?

32. Additional studies show the sensitivity of the 3D mammogram is 94% and the PPV is 98%. You have a patient with a positive 3D mammogram, indicating a high risk of cancer. She wants to know what the chances are that she actually has cancer. What can you tell her?

33. Instead the study design involved looking at 100 women who had both a 2D and a 3D mammogram to determine which screen had higher detection rates. Would a chi-square test be appropriate? Why or why not?

Questions 34–39: In a random sample of patients with oropharyngeal cancer, the researcher wishes to determine if there is a relationship between gender and the type of oropharyngeal cancer. The study has an alpha of 0.05 and a $p = 0.01$.

34. What is the dependent variable?

35. If the type of oropharyngeal cancer is recorded as oral cavity/pharynx, tongue, mouth, pharynx, and other, what level of measurement is this variable?

36. What would be an appropriate test for testing the null hypothesis? Explain.

37. What decision should be made about the null hypothesis? Explain.

38. If this decision is not correct, what potential error could it be?

39. The presence of leukoplakia or erythroplakia in the oropharynx for more than 2 weeks is associated with oropharyngeal cancer. A new tool is developed to screen for oropharyngeal cancer in patients with these symptoms, and it has an NPV of 84%. Your patient's screen is negative, and he wants to know what this means. Explain his result in plain language.

Research Application Article

It is really helpful to start reading professional research articles to see how these concepts are used in actual study scenarios. Give it a try in this article, where the researchers examined the relationship between patients' perception about coffee consumption and distress symptoms in patients with inflammatory bowel disease:

Barthel, C. Wiegand, S., Scharl, S., et al. (2015). Patients' perception on the impact of coffee consumption in inflammatory bowel disease: Friend or foe? A patient survey. *Nutrition Journal, 14*(78). doi:10.1186/s12937-015-0070-8

1. What was the purpose of this study?
2. How are the respondents with inflammatory bowel disease classified?
3. What was the alpha level specified for the study?
4. How many patients with Crohn's disease (CD) responded to the survey? Were they all included in the study?
5. Look at Figure 1 in the article for questions 5–9. How many subjects with CD were included in the study?
6. Which group of patients had the highest percentage who did not drink coffee?
7. Which group had the largest absolute number of patients who did not drink coffee?
8. What percentage of the patients with CD do not drink coffee?
9. What percentage of the sample has CD?
10. Among coffee drinkers, did they prefer caffeinated or decaffeinated coffee?
11. Thirty-eight percent of the sample reported that coffee has an effect on their disease symptoms. Was this the same for the CD and ulcerative colitis (UC) group?
12. Was this difference significant? How do you know?

13. Was the percentage of patients who reported that coffee negatively influenced their intestinal symptoms higher in the CD or UC group? Was this a significant difference? How do you know?

14. Did more of those who felt coffee had a positive impact on their symptoms consume coffee regularly? Was this difference significant? How do you know?

15. What percentage of those who reported a negative effect from coffee still consumed coffee?

16. Look at Figure 3 in the article. Is there a significant difference in the percentage of subjects with CD and UC who report coffee effects their symptoms?

ANSWERS TO ODD-NUMBERED CHAPTER 8 REVIEW QUESTIONS

1. Nominal, categorical

3. Nominal, mode, mode = participating in sports for males and for the total sample

5. H_0: There is no relationship between gender and sports participation

7. See Table 8-8.

TABLE 8-8	Expected Values for Gender and Sports Participation	
	Male	**Female**
No sports	$(80 \times 100) \div 200 = 40$	$(80 \times 100) \div 200 = 40$
Sports participation	$(120 \times 100) \div 200 = 60$	$(120 \times 100) \div 200 = 60$

If your alpha is 0.05, then yes, sports participation is significantly different for males and females. This conclusion is because p is significant.

$$\sum \frac{\left(\text{Observed} - \text{Expected}\right)^2}{\text{Expected}}$$

$$\frac{(30-40)^2}{40} + \frac{(50-40)^2}{40} + \frac{(70-60)^2}{60} + \frac{(50-60)^2}{60}$$

$$100/40 + 100/40 + 100/60 + 100/60 = 8.34$$

$$df = 1$$

9. Type one

11. The outcome variable is nominal/ordinal. It is an independent sample, and the cell values are all >5.

13. Yes, females are more likely.

$df = $ (Number of rows -1) $\times$ (Number of columns -1)
$= 1 \times 1 = 1$

15. Convergent

17. 20 = true positives, 5 = false positives, 10 = false negatives, 215 = true negatives

19. 215/220 = 98%. If the subject does not have the disease, there is a 98% chance the screen will be negative. A specific screen is good at identifying those without the disease.

21. 215/225 = 96%. If the screening test is negative, it is probable that the subject does not have the disease.

23. You would need to use Fisher's exact test because of the small cell size.

25. Type of mammogram, nominal

27. Nominal

29. Fail to reject the null, $p >$ alpha

31. Type two

33. No, these would be dependent samples and would require McNemar's test. Chi-square must have independent samples.

35. Nominal

37. Reject the null, $p <$ alpha

39. Because his screen is negative, we know there is an 84% chance he does not have oropharyngeal cancer.

Research Application Article

Barthel, C. Wiegand, S., Scharl, S., et al. (2015). Patients' perception on the impact of coffee consumption in inflammatory bowel disease: Friend or foe? A patient survey. *Nutrition Journal, 14*(78). doi:10.1186/s12937-015-0070-8

1. To determine if patients with Crohn's disease and ulcerative colitis have different perceptions of the impact of coffee consumption on their disease process

3. Alpha $= 0.05$

5. $209 + 79 = 288$

7. Those with CD. There are 79 patients with CD who do not drink coffee.

9. $288/442 = 65.2\%$

11. No, it was higher for the CD group than the UC group (53.5% versus 22%).

13. The CD group had 45% of subjects who felt coffee worsened their symptoms, while only 20.2% of those with UC reported this finding. It was a significant difference. You know it was significant because $p < 0.001$, which is less than the alpha (0.05) utilized in the study.

15. 49.1%

CHAPTER 9

STUDENT *t*-TEST

HOW CAN I FIND A DIFFERENCE IN THE TWO SAMPLE MEANS IF MY DEPENDENT VARIABLE IS AT THE INTERVAL OR RATIO LEVEL?

OBJECTIVES

By the end of the chapter students will be able to:

- Identify the conditions under which the Student *t*-test is an appropriate statistical technique.

- Compare and contrast dependent and independent samples.

- Identify independent and dependent samples in current nursing research.

- Write null and alternative hypotheses that demonstrate an understanding of the Student *t*-test.

- Calculate the degrees of freedom associated with a given data set.

- Interpret the Statistical Package for the Social Sciences (SPSS) output from a

Student *t*-test, and determine whether it is statistically significant; interpret this result in statistical terms and in plain English; and prepare a public health report using the information.

- Critique an article from current nursing research that utilizes the Student *t*-test, determine what type of sample was collected, identify whether the samples were independent or dependent, determine whether statistical significance is present, and debate whether clinical recommendations should be made.

KEY TERMS

Degree of freedom for *t*-tests
A value that equals the total number of subjects included in both of the comparison groups minus 2.

Dependent samples
Paired or related groups or the same sample at a different time.

Independent samples
Samples that do not have a relationship with one another.

Levene's test for equality of variances
A method that tests the null hypothesis that the variances in the two groups being compared are not different. If Levene's test has a significant *p*-value, you do not assume equal variances. If the Levene's

test does not show a significant *p*-value, you can assume equal variances.

Noninferiority trial
A trial used to show that a new treatment is no worse than an old procedure (may use a one-tailed test).

Sampling error
Error that occurs due to randomization and chance.

Student *t*-test
A test used when you are looking for a difference in the mean value of an interval-level or a ratio-level variable.

THE STUDENT *t*-TEST

One of our favorite statistical tests is called the **Student *t*-test**, which was developed by William Gosset. Before you can apply the Student *t*-test to determine whether there is a difference between the means in two sample groups, you need to determine three things:

- What is the level of measurement for the outcome variable?
- Are there two samples?
- Are the samples independent?

LEVEL OF MEASUREMENT

The Student *t*-test is appropriate only when you are looking for a difference in the mean value of an outcome variable that is at the interval or ratio level. In the "From the Statistician" feature, we look at the difference in the amount of

epinephrine in injectors, which is a ratio-level measurement (i.e., it shows a difference with equal ranked intervals and has a zero value), so it is appropriate.

The next question is, "What kind of samples do you have?" First, are there two samples? To look for a difference in the mean value of the outcome variable, you must have at least two samples. In the epinephrine injector example, you have a sample of injectors from the Acme company and a sample of injectors from the EPI company. So you have two samples, and you are looking for a difference in the mean amount of epinephrine found in each.

Now that you know you have two samples, you have to ask whether how you selected one sample affected the other. In the example, the two samples were randomly collected from two different kinds of injectors without any relationship to each other, so these are two **independent samples**.

FROM THE STATISTICIAN *Brendan Heavey*

Let's Talk *t*-Tests

Fueled by the success of scrubs sales by Carol's Nursing Scrubs, Carol has decided to expand her product offering to include injectable epinephrine pens. Carol has asked you to decide which type of pen she should retail. Two production companies are competing for the job: Acme Pens and EphedraPens International (EPI). They both produce injections that are advertised to hold 0.3 mg of epinephrine. The snag is that both companies have had some bad press recently over the amount of epinephrine in their products. Carol has asked you to check each company and decide whether one type of pen holds more epinephrine than the other.

In this scenario, you're interested in comparing the average amount of epinephrine in Acme's pens with the average amount of epinephrine in EPI's pens—two population parameters. The two companies are not going to give you access to their production facility to test the whole population of pens, so you need to take a sample of each and make some inferences. Obviously, the samples from separate companies are independent of each other.

If it weren't for a man named William Gosset (1876–1937), answering questions like this would be much more difficult. After completing a degree at Oxford in 1899, Gosset decided to do what many other great Celtic men in history did and went to work for the Guinness brewery in Dublin, Ireland. While there, he was enlisted to work on projects to help decide how the quality of hops and barley affected the taste of a "pint o' the black stuff" (the proper way to refer to a glass of Guinness beer in Dublin). After Guinness sent him to study under a great statistician by the name of Karl Pearson, Gosset published a landmark paper that derived the *t*-distribution in 1908. Guinness considered his work top secret, and, as a result, he was forced to publish under the pen name "Student." This is why the *t*-distribution is sometimes referred to as Student's *t* or the Student *t*-test. This test is used when you are looking for a difference in the mean value of an interval- or a ratio-level variable.

Thanks to Gosset's work, we know we can perform an independent samples *t*-test on our epinephrine injection data to determine whether there is a statistical difference between the amounts of epinephrine in the two overall populations of injectors.

Note: All factual information regarding William Gosset was taken from Johnson and Kotz (1997).

However, suppose you collected one sample of Acme injectors, measured their mean epinephrine levels preadministration, gave the injections, and then measured the residual epinephrine levels postadministration to see if there was a difference. (Obviously, if you are injecting the epinephrine there should be!) In that case, you would still have two samples, but they would be **dependent samples**, or related samples. Your second sample is a remeasurement of the same sample group at a different point in time.

You can also have dependent samples when you match sample characteristics. For example, if you are interested in comparing the average duration of hospital stay for individuals at two different hospitals, you might decide you want both samples to have been admitted for the same diagnosis. So you randomly sample 10 patients at the first hospital and measure their length of stay. Then you go to the second hospital and randomly select 10 subjects with the same admission diagnoses as the first group. Now it is important to note that the subjects don't just have a single diagnosis that is the same for everyone in the study (that would be an inclusion criterion); they just share diagnoses equally. For example, if the group from Hospital A has three people with congestive heart failure (CHF), then there has to be three people with CHF in the Hospital B group. If there are 2 people in the hospital A group with a level I head trauma, there must be 2 people selected from the Hospital B group with a diagnosis of a level I head trauma. The two groups are matched on the various diagnoses, but they don't all have the same diagnosis. You could have decided to match the groups for any other criteria you feel is important to control for, such as age. If you had selected to match the groups on age and there were 10 patients ages 45–55 in Hospital A group, then you would select 10 people ages 45–55 in the Hospital B group as well. In either case, because those selected for your second sample must have had the

THINKING IT THROUGH

Tests to consider when comparing two groups and when the outcome variables are at the interval or ratio level:

Sample	Level of Dependent or Outcome Variable	Test	Example
Two independent samples	Interval/ratio	*t*-test for independent samples	Do Asian Americans have a higher mean total cholesterol than African Americans in a random sample of 10,000 Florida state residents? (The independent variable race creates two independent samples to compare; the dependent variable [mean total cholesterol] is interval/ratio.)
Two dependent samples	Interval/ratio	*t*-test for dependent samples	Do husbands and wives have a difference in their mean total cholesterol? (The independent variable husband/wife creates two dependent comparison samples because they are related; the dependent variable [mean total cholesterol] is interval/ratio.)

Note: Samples or groups can be created by the levels of the independent variable. For example, gender may be your independent variable, and the groups you are interested in comparing are men and women, thus creating two samples or groups to compare.

same matching criteria (diagnosis or age) as your first sample, they are not independent samples; they are correlated, or dependent samples. You can still determine whether the average length of stay differs depending on the hospital by comparing the mean from each group; however, to do this accurately, you have to use a *t*-test for dependent groups because you have dependent samples.

In the epinephrine injectors example, however, you know you have an outcome variable that is at the ratio level and two samples that are independent and randomly collected. The presence of these factors means that you can apply the Student *t*-test for independent groups. (Two other factors—normal distribution of the outcome variable and homogeneity of variance—are ideally also present, but they are not absolutely essential, even though they do have an impact on statistical interpretation. You can explore these factors more fully in the "From the Statistician" feature.)

FROM THE STATISTICIAN *Brendan Heavey*

Using a One-Tailed Test

Using a one-sided, or one-tailed, hypothesis test is a controversial procedure that should be avoided in most instances. A researcher who is interested in a *directional* null hypothesis would use a one-tailed test. The assumption is that, based on prior information or previous testing, there is no chance of a change in one of the two possible directions for a particular variable. Therefore, alpha (α), which is usually split between two tails, has its probability shifted to one tail (or one side), as we see in **Figure 9-1**.

One-tailed tests are sometimes acceptable. Their most common use is in **noninferiority trials**, whose point is to show that a new treatment is no worse than an old procedure. For example, a new noninvasive procedure is found that might be a replacement for an older invasive procedure. We don't want to show that the new procedure is better than the old one, only that it is no worse. In this case, using a one-tailed test makes sense because the probability in the *upper* or right side of the tail would indicate that our new noninvasive procedure performed better than our old procedure. Because there is virtually no likelihood of this occurring, we shift the probability to the *lower* or left side of the tail. In this case, we are testing the following null and alternative hypotheses:

H_0: There is no difference between the two therapies.
H_1: The change in response from one therapy is *less than* the change in response from another.

If we were using a two-tailed test, the alternative hypothesis would look like this:

H_1: The change in response from one therapy is different from the change in response from another.

Can you see the difference between these two alternative hypotheses?

(continues)

FROM THE STATISTICIAN *Brendan Heavey*

| FIGURE 9-1 | **Location of Alpha (α) with a Two-Sided versus One-Sided Test.** |

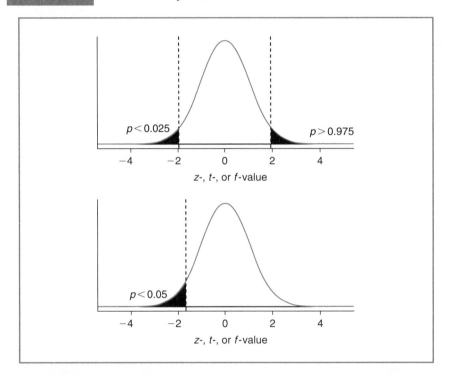

Some researchers overuse one-tailed tests. Why is this practice a problem? Can you figure out why we cannot use one-tailed tests all the time? Is it easier or more difficult to attain statistical significance with a one-tailed test? Let's look at a scenario in which a one-sided test is inappropriate.

Let's say you are working for a pharmaceutical company that has discovered a new drug to treat the flu. The drug is suspected to reduce fever, so your company has you test this hypothesis with the following procedure:

- Enroll 200 subjects who have the flu.
- Administer the test drug to 100 subjects and a placebo sugar pill to the other 100.
- Wait 4 hours and then take everyone's temperature.

FROM THE STATISTICIAN *Brendan Heavey*

In this case, let's say we use a two-sample Student *t*-test to test the difference between average temperatures in these two groups 4 hours after they take the test or placebo pill. You end up with data as shown in **Table 9-1**. The corresponding *p*-value is not significant when we use a two-tailed test, but it is if we use a one-tailed test.

If you are working for the drug company that is pressing to get this new drug to market, you might use a one-sided test based on the argument that there is no chance the new drug will increase fever. Switching to a one-sided test would be a violation of a number of issues, however: You did not decide which test you were going to use beforehand, and you have no prior research to suggest that the pill could not elevate a fever. Needless to say, using a one-tailed test in this situation is not advisable. In fact, one-tailed testing is so frowned upon that some scientific journals require only two-sided *p*-values to be reported. This policy is in place to prevent researchers from cheating and attaining statistical significance in their work too easily.

For examples of appropriate one-sided tests in the literature, see:

- *The Diamond trial:* A noninvasive ultrasound procedure was tested against amniocentesis, an older and more invasive procedure, to test for severe fetal anemia (Oepkes et al., 2006).
- *Neuroblastoma screening:* Researchers investigated whether neuroblastoma screening in infancy improved the survival of children diagnosed with this disease (Schilling et al., 2002).
- *Effect of lidocaine during breast biopsy:* Researchers determined that applying topical lidocaine decreased the pain women experienced during breast biopsy (Olbrys, 2001).

TABLE 9-1	**Clinical Trial for a New Flu Medication**

	Average Temperature after Administration
Drug	101.2
Placebo	102.1

So, before applying an independent Student *t*-test, simply answer the following questions:

- Is my outcome variable at the interval or ratio level?
- Do I have two samples?
- Are my samples random and independent from one another?

If your answers to these three questions are yes, you may proceed with a Student *t*-test for independent groups.

THE NULL AND ALTERNATIVE HYPOTHESES

In the example, the null hypothesis is that there is no difference between the mean amounts of epinephrine in the two types of epinephrine injectors. Our alternative hypothesis, therefore, is that there is a difference between the mean amounts of epinephrine in the two types of pens. We collect our first sample of pens from Acme and find that the average amount of epinephrine in each injector is 0.31 mg. We then collect our second sample of pens from EPI and find the average amount is 0.30 mg. There is a difference in the sample means, but is it statistically significant or is it due to **sampling error** (error that occurs due to randomization and chance)? Because this appears to be a relatively small difference between the means, it is unlikely to be significant, but remember that it could be if the sample size is large.

STATISTICAL SIGNIFICANCE

To determine whether the difference is statistically significant, you have to decide on a number of things:

- *The level of risk you are going to take that you will incorrectly reject the null hypothesis (alpha):* For this example, you decide to take a 5% chance that you will make a type one error, so you select an alpha of 0.05.
- The power (the chance of finding a difference if it actually exists): You decide that 0.80, or 80%, is adequate.
- *Whether you are conducting a one-tailed or two-tailed test:* These terms simply indicate whether you are looking for a difference in either direction (two-tailed) or you have hypothesized that the difference is in a

specific direction, such as the mean in the second sample is greater than or less than the mean in the first (one-tailed). Because this example is looking for a difference in any direction between the epinephrine levels in the two groups, you are going to do a two-tailed Student *t*-test.

DEGREES OF FREEDOM FOR STUDENT *t*-TESTS

This test involves one other concept: **degrees of freedom**, which is equal to the sample size for both groups minus 2. This is the same as taking the degrees of freedom for each group (sample size for the group minus 1) and adding them together. Now you might feel as though you have no freedom, but in your study you do; let's see how much. When you collect a sample of 10 injectors and measure their epinephrine levels, you have 10 values that are "free" to vary depending on which injectors you select and how much epinephrine is in each. However, once you calculate the mean level of epinephrine, only nine of the values are actually free to be "unknown" at any one time. Once you know the amount of epinephrine in each of the nine injector pens and you know the mean, you can figure out how much epinephrine is in the last injector. The value for the last injector pen is no longer free to vary, so when you calculate the mean, you lose a degree of freedom.

If the concept of degrees of freedom still has you totally baffled, just remember this: Take your total sample size (both groups) minus 2 (1 from each group), and you know the degrees of freedom for the test (see **Figure 9-2**). This number is all you need to find the corresponding *p*-value on a *t*-distribution table, which is available in Appendix A. (You can still perform a Student

FIGURE 9-2	**Formula for Calculating Degrees of Freedom for Student *t*-Tests.**

$$\text{Degrees of freedom} = (n_1 + n_2) - 2$$

Where

n_1 = total number of subjects in sample one
n_2 = total number of subjects in sample two

t-test without really understanding degrees of freedom. Just don't tell the statisticians I said so!)

So when are we getting to the really exciting Student *t*-test? The reality of nursing work today is that you won't be making the calculation. However, for those of you who really want to see the equation, you can check it out in the "From the Statistician" feature called Methods: Student's *t*-Test. All the rest of you need only to be able to look at a computer printout or a research article and understand what it means. But wait a minute, you say, when I look at the computer printout for the Student *t*-test, there are two *t*-test values and two *p*-values. What do I do now? Just when we thought SPSS made it so simple, it got confusing for a bit, but don't worry; it isn't so bad. There are two *t* values and two *p*-values, and the one you should report depends on if you can or cannot assume whether the variances in the two groups you are studying are the same. If the variances are the same, the *F* value for the **Levene's test** will be insignificant, and you should report the *t* and *p*-value assuming equal variances. If the variances are not the same, the *F* value for the Levene's test will be significant, and you should report the *t* and *p*-value where equal variances are not assumed. Let's look at an example in **Figure 9-3**.

If we wish to determine if there is a statistically significant difference in the average white blood cell count between patients in an intensive care unit and patients on a medical floor, we need to follow several steps. Using the Figure 9-3, we can see that the Levene's test *F* statistic has a *p*-value $>$ alpha, so we fail to reject the null and assume equal variances in the two samples. But don't be fooled and stop here. We still haven't determined if there is a statistically significant difference in the average white blood cell count (WBC) count in the two groups. We've only determined that the variances between the two groups are about the same.

To determine if there is a statistically significant difference in the average WBC count of the group in the intensive care unit (ICU) and those on a medical floor, we look at the *t* and *p*-value, assuming equal variances. In this example, the *t* value is 2.887 with an associated $p = 0.02$. Because the *p*-value is $<$ alpha, we would reject the null hypothesis (there is no difference in the WBC count between these units). We would conclude there is a difference in the average WBC count of patients in the ICU and in the WBC count of those on a medical floor.

| FIGURE 9-3 | **Independent Samples Test.** |

Independent Samples Test

		Levene's Test for Quality of Variance		t-Test for Equality of Means						
		F	Significance	t	df	Significance (two-tailed)	Mean Difference	Standard Error Difference	95% Confidence Interval of the Difference	
									Lower	Upper
WBC	Equal variance assumed	1.493	.257	2.887	8	.020	2.0000	.6928	.4024	3.5976
	Equal variance not assumed			2.887	6.817	.024	2.0000	.6928	.3528	3.6472

Adapted from statistics-help-for-students.com. (n.d.). How do I interpret data in SPSS for an independent samples T-test? Retrieved from http://statistics-help-for-students.com /How_do_I_interpret_data_in_SPSS_for_an_independent_samples_T_test.htm#.WkvXoCOZOu5

THINKING IT THROUGH

What t-test result do I use?

FROM THE STATISTICIAN *Brendan Heavey*

Methods: Student *t*-Test

Student *t*-test is so named because it makes use of what is called the *t*-statistical distribution. The test is probably the statistical test that is used the most often, for better or worse. I say "for better or worse" because it is not always the correct test to run; it is just usually the most straightforward. The purpose of a two-sample *t*-test is to determine whether the means of two groups differ significantly.

The *t*-test has a few versions, so you have to ask a few questions before performing one:

- *How many tails (one or two) of the statistical distribution do you want to test?* For an in-depth discussion of this topic, see the "From the Statistician" feature called Using a One-Tailed Test earlier in the chapter.
- *Is your data paired?* In some instances, data is set up so that the two groups under consideration have members that are paired instead of being independent. An example of paired data occurs in a so-called crossover clinical trial, in which subjects are given both a placebo and a drug (as shown in **Figure 9-4**). Setting up a trial in this manner is suitable for a paired analysis because each subject has two measures taken: one with the placebo and one with the drug. Because these measures are not measured on two different subjects, the *t*-test that compares their outcomes must be adjusted to account for their nonindependence, and a repeated measures test for the difference in dependent samples should be used.
- *Can you assume equal variances in the two different groups?* One of the assumptions of the two-sample *t*-test is that the two groups have the same variance. Slight departures from this assumption are okay, but if they are too extreme, a different formula should be used. (That alternative is beyond the scope of this text.) Statisticians describe this property as homogeneity of variance or equal variances. (You can try out that vocabulary at your next racquetball match!)

Here is an example of an independent-sample *t*-test to determine if there is a difference in the mean age between two mutually exclusive groups. Data was collected on trauma patients ages 25 and younger during one 72-hour period at an upstate New York tertiary care facility. We were interested in comparing the mean ages between groups who did have a positive drug screen and those who did not. The data set used is shown in **Table 9-2**. We ran a basic analysis in SPSS, whose output is shown in **Tables 9-3** through **9-5** and in Figures 9-4 and **9-5**.

FIGURE 9-4	**Crossover Study Design.**

(continues)

FROM THE STATISTICIAN *Brendan Heavey*

TABLE 9-2	**Age and Drug Screen Status for Patients under Age 25 in a Trauma Center***		
Age	**Drug Screen**	**Age**	**Drug Screen**
2	0	20	0
3	0	20	1
5	0	20	1
7	0	21	1
8	0	22	0
15	1	22	0
15	1	23	1
18	0	23	0
19	0	25	0
19	0	25	0

* Drug screen: 0 = negative, 1 = positive

TABLE 9-3	**Frequency Table for Age**

		Age		
	Frequency	**Percentage**	**Valid Percentage**	**Cumulative Percentage**
Valid 2	1	5.0	5.0	5.0
3	1	5.0	5.0	10.0
5	1	5.0	5.0	15.0
7	1	5.0	5.0	20.0
8	1	5.0	5.0	25.0
15	2	10.0	10.0	35.0

Age				
	Frequency	**Percentage**	**Valid Percentage**	**Cumulative Percentage**
18	1	5.0	5.0	40.0
19	2	10.0	10.0	50.0
20	3	15.0	15.0	65.0
21	1	5.0	5.0	70.0
22	2	10.0	10.0	80.0
23	2	10.0	10.0	90.0
25	2	10.0	10.0	100.0
Total	20	100.0	100.0	

TABLE 9-4 **Descriptive Statistics for Age Variable**

N	Valid	20.0000
	Missing	0.0000
Mean		16.6000
Median		19.5000
Mode		20.0000
Standard deviation		7.4438
Variance		55.4105
Skewness		−0.9158
Standard error of skewness		0.5121
Percentiles	25	9.7500
	50	19.5000
	75	22.0000

(continues)

FROM THE STATISTICIAN *Brendan Heavey*

| TABLE 9-5 | **Means by Drug Screen Status** | | | |

Group Statistics				
Drug Screen		***N***	**Mean**	**Standard Deviation**	**Standard Error Mean**
Age	Negative	14	15.5714	8.54593	2.28400
	Positive	6	19.0000	3.28624	1.34164

| FIGURE 9-5 | **Bar Chart for Age Variable.** |

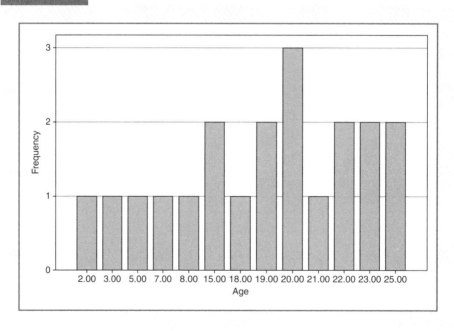

FROM THE STATISTICIAN *Brendan Heavey*

Is the homogeneity of variance assumption appropriate to use in this case? Let's look at the standard deviations of the two groups. We see that the drug-screen-negative group has a standard deviation of 8.54593, whereas the drug-screen-positive group has a standard deviation of 3.28634 (Table 9-5). Tests are available that can be used to decide whether the equivariance assumption holds. The SPSS we chose used Levene's test for equality of variances. Note the large discrepancy in the standard deviations compared to their overall magnitude; we can agree that they are pretty far off from each other. Levene's test for equality of variances tests the null hypothesis that the variances in the two groups are not different. In this example, the Levene's test for equality of variances has a significant p-value, so you reject the null hypothesis that the variances are equal and use the second line of the t-test analysis (for when equal variances are not assumed). That line shows a t-value of -1.294, which converts to a two-tailed p-value of 0.212. Because the study had an alpha of 0.05, you know that this p-value is not adequate to reject H_0. Therefore, you fail to reject H_0: There is not enough evidence to suggest there is a difference in the mean ages of patients in the two groups of a positive and a negative drug screen.

Let's look at a brief computation that explains what makes up the t-value. If the standard deviations for the two groups were similar and we therefore assumed equal variances, you would calculate the appropriate t-value (T) by means of the following formula:

$$T = \frac{\overline{X}_1 - \overline{X}_2}{SE}$$

The difference between the sample means $\overline{X}_1 - \overline{X}_2$ was -3.42857, and the standard error (SE) of the difference, assuming equal variances, was 3.64319; so, the calculation looks like this:

$$\frac{-3.42857}{3.64319} = -0.941$$

Notice that -0.941 is the t-value associated with the test on the statistical computing output table (**Figure 9-6**). If you did not assume equal variances, the denominator would be the standard error of the difference of 2.64, and the resulting t-value would be -1.294 (see Figure 9-6).

(continues)

FROM THE STATISTICIAN *Brendan Heavey*

FIGURE 9-6	t-Test for Equality of Mean Age between Those with a Negative and Those with a Positive Drug Screen.

		Levene's Test for Equality of Variances		t-Test for Equality of Means						
									95% Confidence Interval of the Difference	
		F	Significance	t	df	Significance (two-tailed)	Mean Difference	Standard Error Difference	Lower	Upper
Age	Equal variances assumed	11.098	0.004	−0.941	18	0.359	−3.42857	3.64319	−11.08264	4.22550
	Equal variances not assumed			−1.294	17.960	0.212	−3.42857	2.64889	−8.99459	2.13745

Independent Samples Test

SUMMARY

You have just completed this chapter. Very impressive! Now let's review the main points.

First and most important, remember that the null hypothesis is that there is no difference between the group means. The Student t-test is used to determine whether there is a difference in an interval- or a ratio-level outcome or dependent variable in two sample groups. If the sample groups are independent, the sample groups do not have any relationship. If the samples are dependent, the groups are matched on an attribute or may be the same group measured at a different time; in either case, they are related to each other.

In order to know what t-value and p-value we should report, we first need to determine if the variances in the two groups being examined are equal. Levene's test for equality of variances tests the hypothesis that the variances in the two groups are equal (null hypothesis: no difference in the variances). If Levene's test has a significant p-value, you do not assume equal variances. If the Levene's test p-value is not significant, you can assume equal variances.

Frequently students get as far as determining if the Levene's test is significant but don't complete the next step. Remember, once you know if you can assume equal variances, you apply your decision rule (is p less than alpha?) to the t- and p-values that are either associated with assuming equal variances (if Levene's test is not significant) or those associated with not assuming equal variances (if Levene's test is significant) to determine if you should reject the null hypothesis about variables in your study.

Whew! You made it through another tough chapter. Give yourself a pat on the back and keep in mind how far you have come already! This is tough stuff, but you are getting it!

CHAPTER 9 REVIEW QUESTIONS

Questions 1–11: You are asked to design a study determining whether there is a difference in the average fasting blood glucose for individuals with diabetes randomized either to a strictly dietary intervention or to a diet and exercise intervention.

1. Are you looking for a relationship/association or a difference?

_____

2. What is your dependent variable?

_____

3. Is it qualitative or quantitative? Is it continuous or categorical? What level of measurement is it?

_____

_____

4. How many samples do you have? Is this a probability or nonprobability sampling method?

_____

_____

5. Are these independent or dependent groups?

_____

6. Would you prefer to use a chi-square test or a Student t-test with this study?

_____

7. Write appropriate null and alternative hypotheses.

Null: _____

_____

_____

Alternative: _____

_____

_____

8. Your study includes an alpha of 0.05 and a power of 0.80. You conduct a Student *t*-test, which has a *p*-value of 0.07. What is your conclusion?

_____

_____

9. What type of error might you be making?

10. A trial is repeated with a larger sample, and the Student *t*-test has a *p*-value of 0.04. What is your conclusion now?

_____

_____

11. What type of error might you be making now?

_____

Questions 12–24: Chung and Hwang (2008) examined the difference between an experimental and a control group of patients with leukemia. The experimental group received two follow-up phone calls after discharge, and the control group received routine care. Their Table 2 is reproduced here as **Table 9-6**.

12. What was the independent variable?

_____

| TABLE 9-6 | **Test of Two-Group Differences 4 Weeks after Discharge** |

Variable	Experimental Group (N = 35)		Control Group (N = 35)		t
	X	**SD**	**X**	**SD**	**t**
Self-care	2.67	0.36	1.78	0.38	10.347*
Symptom distress	0.34	0.21	0.82	0.51	5.158*
Quality of life	70.46	18.76	44.15	16.01	6.074*

*$p < 0.001$

Adapted from September 2008 Oncology Nursing Forum article "Education for Homecare patients with Leukemia following a cycle of chemotherapy: An exploratory pilot study" by Yu-Chu Chung, and Huei-Lih Hwang, *Oncology Nursing Forum, 35*(5), pp. E86-E87. Reproduced with permission of the Oncology Nursing Society.

13. What were the dependent variables?

_____

_____

14. What was the mean score for the quality of life for each group?

_____

_____

15. Which group had a higher quality of life 4 weeks after discharge? Was this statistically significant?

_____

_____

_____

16. What was the mean score for self-care for each group?

_____

_____

17. Which group had the ability to provide more of its own self-care? Was this a statistically significant difference?

_____

_____

18. Which group had a higher level of symptom distress? Was this statistically significant?

_____

_____

19. Interpret these findings in plain English, and give a plausible explanation for them.

_____

_____

_____

20. Look at **Table 9-7** from the same study. Interpret the statistically significant results in plain English.

_____

_____

_____

21. Did the experimental group have higher levels of any symptom of distress?

_____

| TABLE 9-7 | **Test of Two-Group Differences of Symptom Distress** |

Variable	Experimental Group ($N = 35$)		Control Group ($N = 35$)		t
	X	SD	X	SD	
Appetite change	1.00	1.59	1.66	1.24	1.931
Fatigue	1.00	0.59	2.11	1.13	5.158***
Appearance change	1.14	1.03	1.54	1.15	1.533
Nausea	0.43	0.61	0.46	0.74	0.464
Irritability	0.29	0.46	0.86	0.73	3.909***
Change in sexual interest	0.71	0.83	1.23	1.17	2.131
Insomnia (sleeplessness)	0.17	0.38	1.09	1.20	4.303***
Dry mouth	0.34	0.48	1.23	1.06	4.502***
Pain	0.37	0.65	0.97	1.22	2.564
Dizziness	0.43	0.65	0.51	0.78	0.498
Lack of concentration	0.23	0.43	0.94	0.87	4.325***
Numbness	0.26	0.44	0.83	0.79	3.748***
Diarrhea	—	—	0.29	0.52	3.260**
Chest discomfort	0.09	0.37	0.43	0.70	2.562*
Oral or esophageal ulcer	0.26	0.44	0.49	0.89	1.364
Stomach discomfort	0.09	0.28	0.23	0.49	1.492
Dyspnea	0.11	0.40	1.02	3.57	1.506
Bleeding	0.11	0.40	0.49	0.92	2.188*
Cough	0.17	0.38	0.60	0.81	2.826*
Trembling	0.09	0.37	0.43	0.74	2.449*
Fever	0.06	0.24	0.40	0.74	2.626*
Dysuria	0.09	0.37	0.14	0.69	0.430

*$p < 0.05$; **$p < 0.01$; ***$p < 0.001$

Adapted from September 2008 Oncology Nursing Forum article "Education for Homecare patients with Leukemia following a cycle of chemotherapy: An exploratory pilot study" by Yu-Chu Chung, and Huei-Lih Hwang, *Oncology Nursing Forum*, 35(5), pp. E86–E87. Reproduced with permission of the Oncology Nursing Society.

22. A convenience sample was used. Is this a probability or nonprobability sampling method?

23. How might this affect the results?

24. How could you improve on this study's sampling method?

Questions 25–31: You are conducting a small study at your hospital looking at infants born in the first 24 hours after the conclusion of a hurricane. You classify prematurity status as full term (0) if the infants are born after 37 weeks of gestation and premature (1) if they are born before 37 weeks of gestation. You measure birth weight in grams at the time of delivery. You conduct a *t*-test to see whether the mean birth weights differ between the premature and full-term infants. See **Table 9-8** and **Figure 9-7**.

25. What is your sample size?

26. What is the mean birth weight for full-term infants?

27. What is the mean birth weight for preterm infants?

28. Which group has a larger standard deviation?

29. Because the Levene's test for equality of variances is not significant, the standard practice is to assume equal variances. What is the appropriate *t*-value?

30. Is the *t*-value significant?

31. What do you conclude?

| TABLE 9-8 | **Mean Birth Weight for Full-Term and Premature Infants** |

Group Statistics				
Preterm Status	**I**	**Mean**	**Standard Deviation**	**Standard Error Mean**
Birth weight 0	6	3453.3333	435.41551	177.75764
1	4	1225.0000	357.07142	178.53571

FIGURE 9-7	*t*-Test for Equality of Mean Birth Weight in Full-Term and Premature Infants.

Independent Samples Test									
		Levene's Test for Equality of Variances		*t*-Test for Equality of Means					
								95% Confidence Interval of the Difference	
		F	Significance	*t*	*df*	Significance (two-tailed)	Mean Difference	Standard Error Difference	Lower	Upper
Birth weight	Equal variances assumed	0.767	0.407	8.465	8	0.000	2228.33333	253.23640	1621.30910	2835.35756
	Equal variances not assumed			7.484		0.000	2228.33333	251.93804	1640.30927	2816.35740

32. "From the Statistician" Review Question: The appropriate *t*-value when not assuming equal variances has been removed from the table in Figure 9-7. Calculate what it would be.

_____

_____

Questions 33–40: A researcher in a Veterans Affairs hospital wants to determine whether patients who had metal-on-metal hardware versus ceramic-on-metal hardware used for their hip replacements have different levels of chromium ions (measured in mcg/mL or parts per billion [ppb] from 0 and up) in their blood 2 years later. A sample of all patients who had full hip replacements with these two types of hardware at the hospital in the last 2 years is collected for a total of 145 subjects in the study. The researcher sets her alpha at 0.05 and her power at 0.80.

33. What is the dependent variable in the study?

_____

34. Serum chromium levels are measured in mcg/mL. What level of measurement is this variable?

_____

_____

35. Would you recommend using a chi-square or an independent *t*-test to answer this question? Why?

_____

36. What type of sample is this? Is it a probability or nonprobability sample?

37. The average serum chromium in the metal-on-metal group is 0.78 ppb, and the average serum chromium in the ceramic-on-metal hardware group is 0.45. The *t*-test results have a *p*-value of 0.043. What conclusion should the researcher draw about the null hypothesis? Why?

38. In this study, the researcher also compares these two groups to see if the type of hardware utilized for the hip replacement results in different average Harris Hip functionality scores 6 months postop (scored from 0–100). What is the independent variable? What level of measurement is this variable?

39. The results in this portion of the analysis have a *p*-value of 0.27. What should the researcher conclude about the null hypothesis for this portion of the study?

40. The researcher later discovers that the effect size for the difference in the Harris Hip functionality is much smaller than she had anticipated. She is now concerned she may have made what type of error in this portion of the study?

Research Application Article

It is really helpful to start reading professional research articles to see how these concepts are used in actual study scenarios. Give it a try in the following article, where the researchers used the *t*-test to analyze the relationship between clinical simulation methodologies and student learning.

Scherer, Y., Foltz-Ramos, K., Fabry, D., & Chao, Y. (2016). Evaluating simulation methodologies to determine best strategies to maximize student learning. *Journal of Professional Nursing, 32*(5), 349–357.

1. This study examined a convenience sample. What does this mean?
2. Group one completes the pretest and posttest knowledge test before and after the simulation experience. The score is measured on a scale of 0–8. What level of measurement is this variable?
3. One of the student groups had their knowledge and performance measures assessed before and after the simulation, then again after repeating the simulation experience a second time. Multiple *t*-tests are utilized to examine the data from two different points in time. Would an independent *t*-test or dependent *t*-test be appropriate to compare the knowledge score on the pretest versus the test after the first simulation?

4. Look at Table 3 in the article. Make sure to read the small print at the bottom of the table. Was there a significant difference between the knowledge scores on the pre- and posttest? How do you know?

5. Look at Table 3 in the article. Was there a significant difference between the knowledge scores on the first posttest and the second posttest?

6. Look at Table 3 in the article. Was there a significant difference in the student's performance measures after repeating the simulation?

7. Look at Table 3 in the article. What was the mean score on the SSSCL on the second posttest?

8. Look at Table 3 in the article. You are asked by the nurse educator to interpret the impact that repeating the simulation had on student satisfaction and self-confidence. What would you report?

9. The study also examined how participation versus observation of the simulation affected student outcomes. Look at Table 4 in the article. What was the average knowledge score on the pretest for the group that was going to participate first (Group A)?

10. Look at Table 4 in the article. What was the average knowledge score on the pretest for the group that was going to observe first (Group B)?

11. Which group of students had a significant change in their own mean knowledge quiz score between the pretest and the first posttest?

12. Look at the measure of the student's self-confidence in the article. Where was there a significant change?

ANSWERS TO ODD-NUMBERED CHAPTER 9 REVIEW QUESTIONS

1. Difference

3. Quantitative, continuous, interval/ratio

5. Independent

7. Answers will vary; for example: H_0: There is no difference in fasting blood glucose in the diet-only group versus the diet and exercise group. H_1: There is a difference in the fasting blood glucose for the two groups.

9. Type two

11. Type one

13. Self-care, symptom distress, quality of life

15. Experimental, yes

17. Experimental, yes

19. Telephone support worked, or the experimental group was just healthier. (They had lower signs and symptoms of distress, and there was nonrandom assignment and no pretest, so we don't know whether this group was healthier at the start.)

21. No

23. The groups may have been significantly different before the intervention.

25. 10

27. 1225 g

29. 8.465

31. Reject the null. There is a significant difference in the mean age of premature infants and full-term infants in this sample.

33. Serum chromium mcg/mL or ppb

35. *t*-test because there are two independent samples and an outcome or dependent variable at the ratio level

37. Reject the null, $p <$ alpha; the metal-on-metal group has a significantly higher average serum chromium level.

39. Fail to reject the null, $p >$ alpha.

Research Application Article

Scherer, Y., Foltz-Ramos, K., Fabry, D., & Chao, Y. (2016). Evaluating simulation methodologies to determine best strategies to maximize student learning. *Journal of Professional Nursing, 32*(5), 349–357.

1. The study included 80 junior nursing students who were enrolled in a particular baccalaureate program. They were not randomized, and they may not reflect the general population of nursing students.

3. Dependent *t*-test. The sample is the same group taking the test both times, which is an example of dependent samples.

5. No, $p = 0.228$, which is greater than the alpha of 0.05.

7. 59.85

9. 4.60

11. Group B. It went from 3.7 to 4.2, and the *p*-value is 0.029, which is less than alpha.

CHAPTER 10

ANALYSIS OF VARIANCE (ANOVA)

HOW DO I COMPARE THE DEPENDENT VARIABLE MEANS FROM MORE THAN TWO SAMPLES?

OBJECTIVES

By the end of the chapter students will be able to:

- Describe the conditions in which ANOVA would be an appropriate test.

- Write null and alternative hypotheses that demonstrate understanding of the guiding principles of ANOVA.

- Determine whether ANOVA test results are significant.

- Describe ANOVA study results in plain English.

- Compare ANOVA and repeat-measures ANOVA.

- Relate situations in which repeat-measures ANOVA would be useful, and explain why.

- Express some limitations or concerns associated with repeat-measures ANOVA.

- Critique a current nursing research article that uses ANOVA, interpret the results statistically and in plain English, and prepare a public health report using this information.

KEY TERMS

Analysis of variance (ANOVA)
The test used when comparing the means from a single dependent variable among two or more groups or samples.

Carryover effect
The condition that occurs when previous treatments continue to have an effect through the next treatment, affecting the measurement of the dependent variable.

Compound symmetry
Measurements are correlated and of equal variances.

Homogeneity of variance
Equal variances among the groups being compared.

Position or latency effect
The condition that occurs when a subject is being exposed to more than one treatment over time, and the order of the treatment received affects the outcome.

Power
Probability of detecting a difference that really exists.

Repeat-measures ANOVA
A test that examines a change over time in the same sample population.

COMPARING MORE THAN TWO SAMPLES

When performing a study, a test is available to find a difference between two groups when you have an outcome variable that is a nominal or an ordinal level of measurement (chi-square test), and another if you have an outcome variable that is an interval or a ratio level of measurement (*t*-test). But both of these methods assume you are examining the differences between only two independent samples. What if you have more than two samples or groups? You could do multiple *t*-tests, but you could compare only two groups at a time, and each comparison would have a risk of a type one error equal to alpha (e.g., 0.05). Even doing three *t*-tests to compare three groups (1 and 2, 2 and 3, 1 and 3) increases the risk of a type one error to 0.05 + 0.05 + 0.05, or 0.15, which is substantial. For this reason, statisticians prefer to use a different test called **analysis of variance (ANOVA)** when comparing more than two groups or sample means.

THE NULL AND ALTERNATIVE HYPOTHESES

Suppose you are working on a study to examine the average systolic blood pressure (SBP) of men from different racial groups. Your sample includes randomly selected male subjects who are Caucasian (group 1), African American (group 2), and Latino (group 3). Your null hypothesis is that all the men will have a similar mean systolic blood pressure regardless of racial background.

$$H_0: \mu_1 = \mu_2 = \mu_3$$

The alternative hypothesis is:

H_1: The three means are not equal.

Note: They don't all have to be unequal. Even if two are significantly unequal, you would reject the null hypothesis.

The analysis of variance test determines whether the differences seen in the sample means are significantly larger than one would expect by mere chance. An equation then produces an *F*-ratio that relates the differences between the groups (the numerator) to the difference within the groups (the denominator). Let's go back to our example for a moment and look at the data we collected to help understand why this matters.

In **Table 10-1** we can see there is variation in the SBP of the subjects in each group. Caucasian men have an SBP that ranges from 110 to 178, African American men have an SBP that ranges from 108 to 196, and Latino men have an SBP that ranges from 110 to 146. We are examining the SBP for 14 different men from each group and wouldn't expect all of them to have the same SBP. The differences we see in the SBP of each subject in an individual group are called the within-group variation.

Now let's look at the average SBP for each group, shown in **Table 10-2**. We can see that African American men have an average SBP of 145.71, which is higher than the average SBP of Caucasian men and the average SBP of Latino men. What we want to determine now is if the differences we see between the groups are any more substantial than the differences we saw within each group. We have to look for the differences between the average SBP

TABLE 10-2	Average SBP for Groups in Our Sample
Racial Group	**Average SBP**
Caucasian	131.57
African American	145.71
Latino	124.71

of each group in relation to the differences we see within each group. If the differences we see between the groups are about the same as the differences we see within the groups, we are more likely to conclude that the null hypothesis is correct and the variation we see is due to chance and not related to the racial background of the subjects. However, if the differences we see between the groups are substantially larger than the differences we see within the groups, we are more likely to reject the null hypothesis and conclude there is an association between racial background and average SBP.

FIGURE 10-1

$$F = \frac{\text{Between Groups Variation}}{\text{Within the Group Variation}}$$

TABLE 10-1	SBP for Caucasian, African American, and Latino Men

Caucasian	134	112	178	156	123	165	110	123	126	118	119	128	132	118
African American	108	196	178	145	164	127	139	142	123	156	150	142	116	154
Latino	110	143	123	120	118	146	124	114	122	116	140	119	130	121

For those of you who are interested, check out the "From the Statistician" feature titled "Methods: Calculating an *F*-Statistic" at the end of the chapter. You can study the details of the equation to your heart's content.

DEGREES OF FREEDOM

As usual, there is also a measure of degrees of freedom. The difference is that the numerator of the *F*-ratio has one number for degrees of freedom (number of groups minus 1), and the denominator of the *F*-ratio has another (the number of subjects minus the number of groups). When you add the two, the sum becomes the degrees of freedom associated with the *F*-ratio.

STATISTICAL SIGNIFICANCE

When the null hypothesis is correct and there is no difference in the means of the groups being studied, the *F*-ratio is close to 1. In that case, the differences between the groups are very similar to the differences within the groups (due to normal individual differences), and the *F*-ratio has an insignificant *p*-value. A larger *F*-ratio value indicates a greater difference when comparing the between-groups variation and the within-groups variation. The larger *F*-ratio is more likely to have a significant *p*-value, but it depends on your sample size, so don't forget to look at the *p*-value to be sure. The *F*-ratio is like any other statistical measure and the *p*-value that determines its significance.

You can look up the *p*-value on a table for the *F*-distribution (see Appendix A), or you can program your statistical computing package to tell you what it is. If the *p*-value is less than the alpha you select (e.g., 0.05), then you have the statistical strength to reject the null hypothesis and report that there is a difference among the averages in the samples or groups. If, on the other hand, you have an alpha of 0.05 and your *F*-ratio has a *p*-value of 0.09, you must fail to reject the null and conclude that you do not have the statistical power to show a difference or that there really isn't one.

Let's consider another example. You conduct a study examining hours of nightly sleep for children, adolescents, and adults and find that the average number of hours slept for children is 10; for adolescents, it is 12; and for adults, it is 6. Your *F*-ratio has a *p*-value of 0.02, and your alpha is 0.05. Because the *p*-value is less than your alpha, you reject the null hypothesis and conclude that there are differences among the average number of hours slept by children, adolescents, and adults. When you report these results, you need to include the means for each group and that there is a statistical difference. But notice that you are not concluding where the statistical difference is located based on your ANOVA results alone.

You cannot conclude from an ANOVA test where the statistically significant difference may lie. Perhaps the average hours slept by children was significantly greater than the average hours slept by adults but not significantly less than adolescents. Perhaps there was a significant difference among all three groups. You would need to do further testing to draw that conclusion. The ANOVA test merely lets you conclude that there is a difference among the average hours of nightly sleep in the three groups.

If you really want to impress people at your next holiday party, show them an analysis of variance test with only two groups (remember, you could do a *t*-test for that!) and then determine the *F*-ratio. If you take the square root, you have the *t*-value, which you could have determined by just doing a *t*-test on the two groups. It is statistically acceptable, but not necessary, to compute an *F*-ratio from an ANOVA test when there are only two groups, and you will reach the same conclusion as you would using the *t*-test. All of this might not be great dinner conversation, but it might come in handy the next time you are trying to discourage a boring date.

APPROPRIATE USE OF ANOVA

Several assumptions should be met before you use ANOVA:

- First, the samples must be independent (ideally random), and the measure must be at the interval or ratio level.

- The sample should have a normal distribution—but remember the central limit theorem. Because we are comparing means, we can comfortably assume normality. The distribution of the original population doesn't matter; the means will be normally distributed.

- The last assumption is **homogeneity of variance**, which also is not terribly concerning at this level because ANOVA still works pretty well even if this assumption is not met.

FROM THE STATISTICIAN *Brendan Heavey*

Relationship between Distributions

What is the relationship among chi-square analyses, *t*-tests, and *F*-tests? The following three facts might surprise you:

- If an ANOVA analysis is performed on just two groups of subjects, the test gives the same results as a *t*-test.
- The *t*-distribution, which is the underlying probability distribution of the *t*-test, looks almost identical to the normal distribution. In fact, the only difference is that it is a little flatter, with more probability assigned to the tails of the distribution.
- An easy way to produce a chi-squared distribution is by summing the squares of a series of standard normal variables.

There are standard ways of converting among these distributions. The math is a bit higher level than we want to discuss here, but it is certainly doable. The process is called *transformation*. Some transformations are quite simple, like the square root transformation performed by taking the square root of every data point in a study variable. Other transformations are quite difficult and can involve formulas longer than a page.

Often, students feel discouraged in introductory statistics classes because they have a difficult time with the properties of distributions and the relationships between them. If you choose to go on to another statistics course (or if you are forced to take another one because of degree requirements), keep in mind the fact that they are all related. Perhaps this insight will give you a bit more motivation to understand their intricacies.

You can choose from an unlimited number of probability distributions. They all must have a total sum of probability, or area under the curve, equal to 1. Whenever you have to deal with a new one, remember the five-step process for statistical testing, and you should be all right. In fact, you can do a surprising amount of decent statistical analysis by learning how to use a basic statistical software package like Statistical Package for the Social Sciences (SPSS). You can thank the great statistical minds that came before us, like Pearson, R. A. Fisher, and Samuel Gosset, for figuring out all the equations for you!

So the big takeaway about assumptions and ANOVA is that you need independent samples with an outcome or a dependent variable at the interval or ratio level. You don't have to be too concerned about the other assumptions. You should know about them, however, because you will see your statistics computing program assess them (Norman & Streiner, 2008).

REPEAT-MEASURES ANOVA

ANOVA has another really exciting application. (I can see you jumping out of your seats with excitement now, but please remain calm!) It is called **repeat-measures ANOVA**, and it is useful for dependent samples. You will see this application used frequently in nursing literature that examines a change over time in the same sample population. For example, suppose you want to compare the mean body mass index (BMI) of a group of children who participated in a 12-week after-school basketball program and a comparison group who did not. BMI becomes your dependent variable, and you are going to measure it, in each of the subjects and the controls, before the subjects begin the program, halfway through the program, and upon completion of the program. You can also design a study appropriate for repeat-measures ANOVA by taking the same group of subjects and measuring their weights before any intervention, then giving them three different weight control interventions, one at a time with 2 weeks per intervention. You then measure their weights before and after each intervention. By repeating the measures on the same group of subjects, you create a level of control over differences among the participants and make it easier to isolate the differences resulting from your

intervention. You thus increase the likelihood that you will find statistically significant results when they exist. In effect, you increase the (can you hear the drum roll here?) **power** of the study (or the ability to detect a difference that really exists). You saw that coming, right?

ISSUES OF CONCERN WITH REPEAT-MEASURES ANOVA

Repeat-measures ANOVA can be very helpful in decreasing not only the individual variation error but also the required sample size needed to find a significant result. This is particularly helpful when it is difficult to recruit subjects or when funding is difficult to obtain. However, all researchers using this method need to be aware of a couple of concerns:

- **Position or latency effects** occur when a subject is being exposed to more than one treatment over time, and the order of the treatment received affects the outcome. For example, let's say you have a cancer study that includes treatment with surgery and chemotherapy. If surgically removing the cancerous tumor improves the ability of the chemotherapy to eliminate any remaining cancer cells, subjects who start with the surgery followed by the chemotherapy may experience a greater effect than those who start with the chemotherapy followed by the surgery. You can address this concern by randomly assigning the order of the interventions.
- **Carryover effects** occur when previous treatments continue to have an effect through the next treatment. In this case, the measurement of the outcome or dependent variable after a particular treatment does not reflect only the impact of that treatment but

THINKING IT THROUGH

When to consider using ANOVA tests:

Sample Type	Level of Dependent or Outcome Variable	Test	Example
Two or more independent groups or samples	Interval/ratio	ANOVA	Is there a difference in the mean body mass index (BMI) among nurses who work days, evenings, or nights? (The independent variable creates three independent samples to compare [shift worked]. The dependent variable of BMI is at the interval/ratio level.)
One group with outcomes measured at multiple points over time	Interval/ratio	Repeat-measures ANOVA	Is there an improvement in a general knowledge score for a sixth-grade class given a pretest, then an educational intervention, followed by a 6-week posttest and a 12-week posttest? (Only one group with the dependent variable or outcome of an interval/ratio test score is measured at multiple points over time.)

Note: Samples or groups can be created by the levels of the independent variable. For example, marital status may be your independent variable, and the groups you are interested in comparing are married, divorced, living together, and single, which creates four samples or groups to compare.

also includes the additional effect from the previous treatment. For example, if subjects in a weight study take a diet pill with a long half-life, they may need a "washout" period before beginning the next intervention to avoid having the effect of two interventions at the same time (Plichta & Garzon, 2009).

APPROPRIATE USE OF REPEAT-MEASURES ANOVA

Like all other statistical techniques, appropriate use of repeat-measures ANOVA involves meeting some basic assumptions. Most of the assumptions are the same as those for ANOVA, but there is one more—**compound symmetry**. Compound symmetry means that the measurements are correlated and of equal variances. If you are measuring BMI three times, the three results should be correlated with one another and be approximately the same. Homogeneity of variance, the term used to indicate that those correlated BMI measurements need to have approximately equal variances, should also be present.

The good news is that, once again, your statistical computing package will check all of this for you. If you look at your SPSS output, you will see an area for Mauchly's sphericity test. If this test is not significant, you can tell the assumption of compound symmetry is met and can proceed with your analysis confidently (Munro, 2005). What on earth did we do before SPSS? Okay, I have to admit, I remember—and it wasn't pretty.

FROM THE STATISTICIAN   *Brendan Heavey*

Methods: Calculating an *F*-Statistic

An analysis of variance is a lot like a *t*-test extended to multiple groups of data. It is a little more difficult to understand conceptually, but in my opinion, it is well worth the effort to learn! In fact, if you don't use ANOVA, you sometimes have to do a whole series of *t*-tests, and that can quickly increase the error associated with your analysis.

Let's say we have two variables: One is continuous, and one is categorical. The categorical variable has three levels, and we are interested in looking at the mean value of the continuous variable in each of these categories. (See **Table 10-3**.) Each of the three cells in the table has its own mean, which is identified using the Greek letter μ (mu). (Don't ask me why we use ancient Greek; we follow the mathematicians' lead on this.) Attached to each μ character is a subscript that indicates the number of the group from which the mean is determined. The overall mean (or grand mean) is denoted by a period ($\mu.$). In ANOVA, we are always interested in a null hypothesis that makes all of the individual cell means equal to one another.

To perform a test of this hypothesis, we compute an *F*-statistic (named after R. A. Fisher, who developed ANOVA). The *F*-statistic is simply a ratio of variances. (Remember, variance is a measure of how a set of values differs from a single value.) The first variance component in an *F*-statistic is derived from the variance of the cell means around the grand mean. (This is the variance between the groups.) The second variance component in an *F*-statistic is derived from how each individual data point differs from its respective cell mean. (This is the variance within the group itself.)

Let's look at an example. We collected data on trauma cases ages 25 and younger during one 72-hour period at an upstate New York tertiary care facility. We then compared the mean age between groups who had a positive drug screen and those who did not. Now we are interested in seeing whether the mean age of a patient differs among the classes of injury for which the patients had been treated. The data is presented in **Table 10-4**.

The first step is to get our data to look like the generalized table in **Table 10-5**. **Table 10-6** shows how our data looks in the general ANOVA table.

Now we solve for the unknown parameters:

$$\mu_1 = \frac{5+25}{2} = 15$$

$$\mu_2 = \frac{7+19+20+23+23}{5} = 18.4$$

$$\mu_3 = \frac{2+3+8+15+15+18+19+20+20+20+22+22+25}{13} = 16.08$$

$$\mu. = \frac{5+25+7+19+20+23+23+2+3+8+15+15+18+19+20+20+20+22+22+25}{20} = 16.6$$

In this hypothesis, our null hypothesis is: H_0: The three *cell means* are equal.

FROM THE STATISTICIAN *Brendan Heavey*

TABLE 10-3	**Beginning of General ANOVA Table**			
	Level 1	**Level 2**	**Level 3**	**Grand Mean**
Variable	μ_1	μ_2	μ_3	$\mu.$

TABLE 10-4 — **Age and Injury Level for Patients Seen in a 72-Hour Period at a Trauma Center**

Age	Injury	Age	Injury
2	2	20	1
3	2	20	2
5	0	20	2
7	1	20	2
8	2	22	2
15	2	22	2
15	2	23	1
18	2	23	1
19	1	25	0
19	2	25	2

TABLE 10-5 — **Setting Up a General ANOVA Table for Age and Injury Example**

	Factor Level 1	**Factor Level 2**	**Factor Level 3**	**Grand Mean**
Variable	μ_1	μ_2	μ_3	$\mu.$

TABLE 10-6 — **Our Data in the General ANOVA Table**

	No Injury	**Minor Injury**	**Major Injury**
Age	5, 25	7, 19, 20, 23, 23	2, 3, 8, 15, 15, 18, 19, 20, 20, 20, 22, 22, 25

(continues)

FROM THE STATISTICIAN *Brendan Heavey*

The alternative hypothesis is: H_1: They are not *all* equal.

The results of the ANOVA are shown in **Table 10-7**. The p-value for this test is 0.815, derived from the F-statistic value of 0.207. Assuming an alpha of 0.05, this p-value indicates that there is not enough evidence to reject the null hypothesis.

Where does the F-statistic value come from? It is the mean square between groups divided by the mean square within groups or, using data from Table 10-7:

$$F = \frac{12.414}{60.007} = 0.207$$

Where do the mean squares come from? These are the sums of squares divided by their respective degrees of freedom. Look at Table 10-7, and you can see that the following is true:

$$\frac{24.827}{2} = 12.414 \quad \frac{1020.123}{17} = 60.007$$

Now we come to the big question: Where do the sums of squares come from? They are the measurements of the variance components from two different sources:

- How much the cells' means vary around the grand mean
- How much the individual data points vary around their respective cell means

The analysis of variance compares these two measures to derive the F-statistic.

If you want to see ANOVA in action, check out the articles by Chen, Shiao, and Gau (2007); Papastavrou et al. (2009); and Zurmehly (2008).

TABLE 10-7   **Statistical Program Output: ANOVA Table**

Age	ANOVA				
	Sum of Squares	**df**	**Mean Square**	**F**	**p-value**
Between groups	24.8269	2	12.4135	0.2069	0.815
Within groups	1020.1231	17	60.0072		
Total	1044.9500	19			

Summary

You are doing a spectacular job at learning these concepts if you made it this far! Let's review the main points from this chapter.

The analysis of variance (ANOVA) is used when comparing the sample means for a single dependent variable among two or more independent groups or samples. An ANOVA test produces an F-ratio with a corresponding p-value. The F-ratio compares the variation between the group means to the variation seen within the groups. If the associated p-value is less than alpha, you reject the null and conclude that there is a difference in the sample means in the groups studied. Further testing is required to identify where the statistically significant difference is located.

The repeat-measures ANOVA is used to examine a change over time in the same sample population. The test is useful for dependent samples. When using repeat-measures ANOVA, you must be aware of position or latency effects. These effects can occur when a subject is being exposed to more than one treatment over time, and the order of the treatments received can have an impact on the outcome in different ways. Also, be aware of carryover effects, which occur when previous treatments continue to have an effect through the next treatment, and the measurement of the dependent variable may not be accurate.

CHAPTER 10 REVIEW QUESTIONS

Questions 1–12: In a study by Vassiliadou et al. (2008), the role of nursing in sexual counseling of myocardial patients was examined. The authors examined professional nurses and collected data about their gender, age, education, unit of employment, and experience in cardiac clinics. They then compared, among other things, the knowledge and comfort level nurses had with regard to sexual counseling.

Vassiliadou, A., Stamatopoulou, E., Triantafyllou, G., Gerodimou, E., Toulia, G., & Pistolas, D. (2008). The role of nurses in the sexual counseling of patients after myocardial infarction. *Health Science Journal, 2*(2), 111–118. Reprinted with permission from *The Health Sciences Journal*.

1. What are the dependent variables?

2. Knowledge is measured by the score in points that the nurse receives on a test. Is this a quantitative or qualitative variable? Is it continuous or categorical? What level of measurement is it?

3. These researchers conducted surveys at a nursing conference. What type of sample is this? How does this affect the generalizability of the results?

4. Write an appropriate null hypothesis.

5. Write an appropriate alternative hypothesis.

6. The study has an alpha of 0.05 and a power of 80%. The researchers found a relationship between the unit that the nurses worked on and the knowledge scores, with a p-value of 0.01. What should the researchers conclude?

7. When comparing nurses from different units and their comfort with this type of counseling, the researchers found a p-value of 0.17. What should they conclude about the comfort level of nurses from different units?

8. Comparing nurses from different units and their comfort level with this type of counseling yielded a p-value of 0.17. What is the F-value probably close to?

9. If this conclusion is incorrect, what type of error would the researchers be making?

10. What is the probability of making this type of error?

11. If the researchers think this type of error is occurring, what might they do to fix it?

12. Why is ANOVA an appropriate test for this study?

Questions 13–21: A study by Heyman et al. (2008) examined a sample of 245 elderly individuals living in long-term care facilities. Each had a grade II–IV pressure ulcer. The pressure ulcers were examined at enrollment and then again at 3 and 9 weeks. All of the patients received standard care plus an additional nutritional supplement. The goal of the study was to examine the effects of the nutritional supplement plus routine care on the healing of pressure ulcers in long-term care patients. (See **Figure 10-2.**)

FIGURE 10-2	**Reduction in Mean Pressure Ulcer Area Achieved with the Oral Nutritional Supplement.**

Mean data ± SE

* $p < 0.0001$ Compared with baseline; ^ $p < 0.0001$ compared with week 3, visit 2

13. What is the dependent variable?

14. What is the independent variable?

15. What level of measurement is the dependent variable?

16. Is it qualitative or quantitative?

17. Is it continuous or categorical?

18. Is the sample independent or dependent?

19. All subjects who met eligibility requirements and consented to treatment at 61 long-term care facilities were enrolled, with no exclusion criteria. What type of sampling method is this?

20. Write an appropriate null hypothesis.

21. Write an appropriate alternative hypothesis.

Questions 22–31: Look at Figure 10-2.

22. This study has an alpha of 0.05 and a power of 0.80. Was the size of the pressure ulcer at the first follow-up (visit 2) significantly different from the size at visit 1?

23. Was the size of the pressure ulcer significantly different at the 9-week follow-up (visit 3)?

24. What would you conclude regarding your null hypothesis?

25. What type of error could you be making?

26. What is your chance of making this type of error?

27. As the nurse manager in a long-term care facility, you believe these results are clinically significant. What recommendation would you make in terms of clinical care?

28. Why is repeat-measures ANOVA an appropriate choice for analysis?

29. By using this sample as their own control group, these researchers were able to minimize the effect of differences among the participants and see the effect of the intervention more clearly. What did this increase in the study?

30. Using the participants as their own controls minimized the effect of the differences among the participants. How does this affect the sample size needed?

31. Any researcher using repeat-measures ANOVA needs to be aware of position and carryover effects. What are these? Are they a concern in this study?

32. "From the Statistician" Review Question: You are asked to evaluate a nursing program's admission criteria and want to determine whether the mean grade point average (GPA) is different for individuals with higher-ranked letters of recommendation (on a five-point scale: 1 = poor, 5 = excellent). You develop the following ANOVA table:

ANOVA

GPA					
	Sum of Squares	**df**	**Mean Square**	**F**	**Significance**
Between groups	0.686	4			0.316
Within groups	12.122	85			
Total	12.807	89			

Complete the calculations necessary to fill in the rest of the table. What do you conclude?

Questions 33–45: The owners of a large clothing manufacturing plant are considering enacting a footwear policy for employees and have started to gather data on the type of foot coverage worn and injuries. When employees sign in for their shift, they now have to indicate the type of foot coverage they are wearing. The occupational health nurse on site believes there is an association between foot injuries and the type of foot coverage worn by the employees in the plant. The nurse decides to evaluate the average number of foot injuries in those wearing open-toed shoes, closed-toed shoes, and steel-toed boots and selects an alpha of 0.05 and a power of 0.80. She is also concerned because the plant has two separate buildings, and she wants to make sure her sample is representative of the population and includes equal representation from both buildings.

33. Write appropriate null and alternative hypotheses.

_____

_____

34. What is the dependent variable?

_____

_____

35. What level of measurement is the dependent variable?

_____

_____

36. What test would you use to compare these groups? Why?

_____

_____

37. The nurse divides the population based on the building the employees work in and then randomly selects 50% of the sample from each building for a total of 1,000 subjects in her sample. She then reviews the files of these employees to assess the number of foot injuries and the type of footwear worn at the time of injury in the last 10 days. What type of sample is this? Is it a probability or nonprobability sample?

_____

_____

38. After collecting the data, the nurse creates a bar chart to present the data. What should be on the horizontal and vertical axes in this chart?

39. The nurse finds the following:

Foot Covering	Average Number of Injuries in 10 Days
Open toe	1.47
Closed toe	1.12
Steel toe	0.01

The nurse also wishes to present a grouped frequency table to illustrate the difference in the frequency of injury in steel-toed footwear ($n = 1/211$) versus non-steel-toed footwear ($n = 42/313$) for the whole population of employees at the plant on the last day of the study ($N = 524$). Show the results.

40. When the nurse analyzes her data, she completes an ANOVA comparing the average number of injuries in each of the three groups, and her F-value is $p = 0.001$. What decision should she make about the null? Why?

41. Interpret this result in plain English. Does the nurse know where the statistically significant difference is?

42. The nurse would like to support her argument that all employees should wear steel-toed boots. She now wants to compare the population data for injuries in steel-toed versus non-steel-toed footwear. What would be an appropriate test to use in this situation? Why?

43. The nurse completes her analysis comparing steel-toed versus non-steel-toed footwear and injuries. Her p-value is 0.00017. What should she conclude about the null hypothesis? Why?

44. Look at the grouped frequency data and the significant p-value found in the nurse's t-test to compare the steel-toed versus non-steel-toed footwear. Which group is more likely to experience foot injuries?

45. The nurse presents her results at a national conference, where the clinical experts in the field agree these results are critically important to employee health. Are these results clinically significant? Why or why not?

Research Application Article

Let's look at the use of ANOVA in the following nursing research article:

Özden, D., & Görgülü, R. S. (2015). Effects of open and closed suction systems on the haemodynamic parameters in cardiac surgery patients. *Nursing in Critical Care, 20*(3), 118–125. doi:10.1111/nicc.12094

1. What was the purpose of the study? What were the independent and dependent variables?
2. What level of measurement was the independent variable?
3. What level of measurement were the dependent variables?
4. Why does this study matter to evidence-based practice?
5. The authors report that they found several studies during their literature review that reported significant differences between utilizing open and closed suction systems; however, these differences were small and clinically irrelevant. What does this statement tell you about the statistical and clinical significance of the studies in question?
6. This study was conducted in a cardiovascular surgery intensive care unit (CVS-ICU) in Turkey that utilized both open and closed endotracheal suction (ES). What were the inclusion criteria for the study?
7. What were the exclusion criteria?
8. Of the 258 patients admitted during the time frame of the study, the researchers selected 120 from a list of previously designated surgical patients. This is an example of what type of sampling method?
9. What do you know about the demographic characteristics of the two groups? Were the demographics of the two groups similar?
10. When were the hemodynamic parameters measured?
11. How does repeating and comparing the hemodynamic measures on the same subjects over time affect the power of the study?
12. Look at Table 1 in the article. Which group had a higher PaO_2 level before any intervention at all? Was this a significant difference?
13. What happened to the average PaO_2 level for patients who had open ES from baseline to as soon as the suctioning was terminated?
14. Look at Table 1 in the article. What happened to the average PaO_2 level for patients who had closed ES from baseline to as soon as the suctioning was terminated?
15. Look at Table 1 in the article. The researchers compared the PaO_2 levels for patients as soon as the suctioning was terminated using a *t*-test. What did they report?
16. Look at Table 1 in the article. What happens to the average PaO_2 level in the open ES group over time?
17. Look at Table 1 in the article. What happens to the average PaO_2 level in the closed ES group over time?'
18. Look at Table 1 in the article. Were the differences in the average PaO_2 level in the two groups significant at any single point of measure?
19. Look at Table 1 in the article. The researchers looked at the average PaO_2 level within the open ES group at multiple points in time utilizing repeat-measures ANOVA. What does this test result indicate?
20. If the researchers had compared the groups only to each other and not to themselves, what impact could this have had on the results?
21. Look at Table 1 in the article. The researchers looked at the average PaO_2 level within the closed ES group at multiple points in time utilizing repeat-measures ANOVA. What does this test result indicate?
22. The researchers report that they completed a post hoc *t*-test and evaluated the average PaO_2 level for patients who had open ES from baseline to as soon as the suctioning was terminated. Was it significant?

23. Was the average PaO_2 level immediately after ES significantly different from the average PaO_2 level at other points in time in both groups?
24. How do the researchers explain these results?
25. If the researchers had missed the significance of the drop in the average PaO_2 level within the open ES group, what type of error would this be?

ANSWERS TO ODD-NUMBERED CHAPTER 10 REVIEW QUESTIONS

1. Knowledge and comfort level

3. Nonprobability convenience sample; may not be representative; may be a more educated group of nurses or a particularly interested group of nurses

5. Answers will vary; for example, H_1: There is a difference in the knowledge level of nurses working on different units.

7. Fail to reject the null; there is no significant difference.

9. Type two

11. Increase the sample size

13. Pressure ulcer size

15. Collected as ratio-level data, analyzed as ordinal-level data

17. Continuous

19. Nonprobability; convenience sampling

21. Answers will vary; for example, H_1: Pressure ulcers decrease in size by 9 weeks.

23. Yes

25. Type one

27. To give the nutritional supplement

29. Power

31. Position effects (if the order of the interventions affects the outcome) can be avoided by random assignment, and carryover effects need a washout period. Because this study had only one intervention, these are not a concern.

33. Null: There is no relationship between type of foot coverage worn and foot injuries. Alternative null: The average number of foot injuries for those in open-toed, closed-toed, or steel-toed shoes is the same.

35. Ratio

37. Stratified, probability sample

39.

Type of Footwear	Number of Injuries in the Last 48 Hours
Non-steel-toed ($n = 313$)	42
Steel-toed ($n = 211$)	1

41. There is a statistically significant difference among the number of foot injuries in the three groups; however, the nurse cannot determine where the statistically significant difference actually is without further analysis.

43. Reject the null, $p <$ alpha.

45. Yes, it is clinically significant because it is statistically significant, and the experts in the field agree it is clinically important as well.

Research Application Article

1. To examine the impact of open and closed suction systems on the hemodynamic status of patients after open heart surgery. The independent variable was the type of suctioning system utilized, and the dependent variables were heart rate (HR), mean arterial pressure (MAP), oxygen saturation (Spo$_2$), and blood gases.

3. Ratio

5. The study found statistically significant results that were not clinically significant.

7. Those re-operated on for revision, those who received inotrope or vasoactive drugs, and those who had ES performed during the first 4 hours post-op were not included.

9. The open ES group was 71.7% male and had an average age of 56.2 years; the closed ES group was 53.3% male and had an average age of 54.9 years, with a higher standard deviation as well. The demographics are not matched and do contain differences, which could have an impact on the outcomes.

11. It increases the power or ability to find a difference that really exists because it minimizes the variance among different participants and allows you to further identify the difference associated with the intervention itself.

13. It dropped from an average of 134.67 to124.54.

15. They reported a *t*-value of 0.601, which is not significant ($p = 0.549$).

17. It increases at all points, including during ES, and climbs to a level higher than baseline over time, indicating signs of improved oxygenation.

19. The *F*-statistic is 10.688 with a corresponding *p*-value of 0.00, which means that there are significant differences in the average PaO$_2$ level within the open ES group over time.

21. The *F*-statistic is 1.49 with a corresponding *p*-value of 0.22, which means that there are no significant differences in the average PaO$_2$ level within the open ES group over time.

23. The average PaO$_2$ level immediately after ES was significantly different from the average PaO$_2$ level at other points in time when open ES was utilized but not when closed ES was utilized.

25. A type two error, missing an association that really exists

CHAPTER 11

CORRELATION COEFFICIENTS

HOW CAN WE LOOK FOR A RELATIONSHIP BETWEEN TWO VARIABLES IN THE SAME GROUP?

OBJECTIVES

By the end of this chapter students will be able to:

- Identify situations in which using a correlation coefficient is appropriate.

- Compare correlation coefficients, and determine when the requirements of each are met.

- Appropriately match the level of measurement of a variable and the appropriate correlation coefficient test.

- Write null and alternative hypotheses that demonstrate an understanding of the guiding principles of correlation coefficients.

- Evaluate a correlation coefficient, and assess the direction of the relationship.

- Differentiate between the strength and the direction of the relationship.

- Determine whether a correlation is statistically significant.

- Identify and calculate the percentage of variance.

- Explain in plain English what the percentage of variance means, and prepare a public health headline using this information.

- Read and interpret a computer printout with correlation coefficients, identify whether the correlation coefficient is statistically significant, identify the direction of the relationship and the strength of the relationship, and state these results in statistical terms and in plain English.

- Critique a current nursing research article that uses correlation coefficients, interpret the results statistically and in plain English, and prepare a public health report using this information.

KEY TERMS

Chi-square test
The test used to find a relationship or difference in an outcome or a dependent variable measured at the nominal or ordinal level.

Coefficient of determination
The square of Pearson's r (r^2).

Correlation
A relationship between at least two variables.

Direction of the relationship
Either the positive or the negative nature of the relationship. If positive, both variables move in the same direction; if negative, one variable increases in value when the other decreases, and vice versa.

Homoscedasticity
Equal spread of one variable around all the levels of another variable.

Pearson's correlation coefficient (r)
The test used if you are looking for a relationship between two variables that are normally distributed and are at the interval or ratio level.

Percentage of variance
The amount of variance in one variable that is explained by the second variable. It is determined by multiplying the coefficient of determination by 100.

Spearman correlation coefficient (ρ)
The test used to determine whether there is a relationship between two variables that are ordinal, interval, or ratio level but don't meet the full assumptions for use of the Pearson's correlation coefficient (such as normality of distribution).

Strength of the relationship
Determined by the absolute value of the correlation coefficient.

LOOKING FOR A RELATIONSHIP IN ONE SAMPLE

Sometimes nurses want to know the relationship or association between two variables in a single group. For example, is there an association between working overtime hours and medication errors among the nurses in your hospital? You'll notice in this example that there is no comparison group; rather, there is simply a question about the relationship or correlation between the two variables.

THE NULL AND ALTERNATIVE HYPOTHESES

In this example, you would develop the following null and alternative hypotheses.

H_0: There is no association between overtime hours worked and medication errors.

H_1: There is an association between overtime hours worked and medication errors.

When they did this very study in New York, they found a statistically significant positive relationship between overtime hours worked and medication errors, so they rejected the null hypothesis. The public health laws were changed as a result, and it is now illegal in New York State to mandate a nurse to work overtime beyond a 16-hour shift. Nurses who work shifts longer than this voluntarily (or for the extra income) are held personally responsible for any errors they make due to fatigue or exhaustion (New York State Nurses Association, n.d.). This is an example of looking for a relationship, or **correlation**, between two variables—in this case, hours worked and medication errors.

SELECTING THE BEST CORRELATION TEST TO USE

For the several types of correlation tests, the lead question is the same as it was before: What level of measurement are my variables? Now you can understand why this is such an important question in statistics! The level of measurement of the variables involved in any analysis affects what you can do with the data and what conclusions you can draw. If you are looking for a relationship between categorical variables (nominal or ordinal, which are treated like nominal variables using this test) in a single sample, you can use the **chi-square test** from Chapter 8 (what a flexible test). However, if you are looking for a relationship between variables that are at least at the ordinal level, follow these general guidelines:

- If the lowest level of data collected for at least one of the variables is measured at the ordinal level or is not normally distributed, you should use the **Spearman correlation coefficient (ρ)** (the Greek letter rho). (You can sometimes use the Pearson's correlation coefficient with ordinal data too, but that is a long story, and you don't need to worry about it now.)
- If you have two variables that are at the interval or ratio data level and they are normally distributed, you can use the **Pearson's correlation coefficient (r)**.

DIRECTION OF THE RELATIONSHIP

Both the Spearman and Pearson's correlation coefficients describe the direction and strength of a linear relationship between two variables. A linear association is represented by a straight line. The **direction of the relationship** is either positive or negative. A positive correlation means that when one variable increases, the other variable does too, and when one decreases, so does the other. Both variables move in the same direction. In a positive correlation, the coefficient (ρ or r) is positive. Let's use every professor's favorite example of a positive relationship. The relationship between the time spent studying for an exam and the grade received on the exam is usually positively correlated. (Yes, we do this for subliminal messaging effect as well.) Conversely, if less time is spent on studying, the grade received is usually lower.

In a negative relationship or correlation, if one variable increases, the second variable decreases, and vice versa. For example, the relationship between smoking and life expectancy has a negative correlation. When smoking increases, life expectancy decreases; when smoking decreases, life expectancy increases. In this case, the correlation coefficient (ρ or r) is negative.

SAMPLE SIZE

You must have a sample of at least three subjects for correlation coefficients. If you are looking for a linear relationship between only two measures (subjects) of a variable, you will always find one: You can always connect two points with a straight line (that's why it is called linear). For all of these tests, you need two variables to correlate and at least three subjects in the sample; then you can compute the appropriate correlation coefficient.

STRENGTH OF THE RELATIONSHIP

The **strength of the relationship** or correlation is determined by the absolute value of the correlation coefficient. Absolute value is just the numeric value of a number without the positive or negative indicator. For example, the absolute value of -4 is 4, and the absolute value of $+4$ is 4.

Correlation coefficients are always between -1 and 1.

- A correlation coefficient of -1 indicates a perfect negative relationship.
- The closer the correlation is to 0, the weaker the relationship is.
- If the correlation is 0, there is no relationship at all. In this case, the variables are completely independent.
- At the other extreme, a correlation coefficient of 1 indicates a perfect positive relationship.

- If the *absolute* value of the correlation coefficient is < 0.3, the relationship between the variables is weak.
- If it is 0.3–0.5, the relationship between the variables is moderate.
- If it is > 0.5, the relationship between the variables is strong.

For example, putting the direction and strength concepts together, a correlation coefficient of 0.2 shows a weak positive relationship between the variables. A correlation coefficient of -0.6 shows a strong negative relationship between the variables.

STATISTICAL SIGNIFICANCE

But wait a minute here—do not be fooled. You need to look at something else to determine whether these results are significant. What do you always need to check before you know whether the results are statistically significant? *Yes*—the *p*-value! Your statistical computing package will give you a corresponding *p*-value, which determines whether your correlation coefficient is significant. If your sample size is very small, you may have large correlation coefficients that are not significant ($p >$ alpha). Even small correlation coefficients can be significant when the sample is large ($p <$ alpha).

Nurses usually remember this quite well. I usually remind my class that the last step at the end of a nursing shift (tabulating the patient's intake and output for the shift) and the last step at the end of a statistics test are remarkably similar. You always have to check the "pee" value! You have to know the *p*-value before you are done with your statistical analysis as well.

Appropriate Use of Correlation Coefficients

Selecting any test depends on certain assumptions, which for correlation coefficients should include the following:

- First, the sample subjects should be independent and randomly selected.
- Second, the level of measurement for each variable should be identified and utilized for selecting the appropriate correlation coefficient.
- Third, two variables must be compared, and a linear relationship must be present. (You can always check a scatterplot to make sure this is the case.)
- If you wish to use the Pearson's correlation coefficient, both variables should be normally distributed in the population (the fancy term for this is *bivariate normal*), and **homoscedasticity** should be present.

  Homoscedasticity can be seen visually on a scatterplot. It is a truly horrific word to try to say, but its meaning is pretty simple. If the spread of a variable is about the same around all the levels of another variable, this assumption is met. For example, if one to two more nursing errors occur for each additional hour of work, homoscedasticity is present. However, if at 5 hours of work, 0 to 3 more errors occur; at 10 hours of work, 0 to 9 more errors are reported; and at 15 hours of work, 1 to 15 more errors are reported, this assumption is violated. These last two assumptions for the Pearson's correlation coefficient can be violated if the sample size is large enough. The big takeaway about these assumptions is to make sure that your sample has at least 50 subjects. Then you can proceed as long as you have ratio-/interval-level data (Corty, 2007).

Here are some questions to answer before you select the best correlation test:

- Do you have one independent group and no comparison group as your sample?
- Are you looking for a linear relationship between two variables in this sample?
- What is the lowest level of measurement for each of your variables?
  - *Two nominal variables:* Select chi-square.
  - Ordinal and ordinal/interval/ratio variables: Select Spearman's.
  - *Both variables are interval/ratio and meet Pearson's assumptions:* Select Pearson's.
  - *Both variables are interval/ratio but do not meet Pearson's assumptions:* Select Spearman's.

When selecting the correlation test, make sure that your data meets the test's assumptions. If it does not, you need to select a test at a lower level. For example, if you wish to use Pearson's correlation coefficient but your sample is only 20 subjects and is not normally distributed, you generally need to use the Spearman's correlation coefficient.

More Uses for Pearson's *r*

You should know one other thing about the Pearson's *r*. If you square it (r^2), it becomes the **coefficient of determination**. If you then multiply it by 100, it tells you something called the **percentage of variance**, which nurses readily understand. The percentage of variance is simply the amount of variance in one variable that is explained by the second variable.

For example, suppose you were reading a study that found that daily caloric intake and total serum cholesterol had a statistically significant Pearson's correlation coefficient of 0.7 ($r = 0.7$). You could square this number ($0.7 \times 0.7 = 0.49$) to calculate the coefficient of determination. When you multiply that coefficient by 100, you can then use plain English again: "Forty-nine percent of the differences they found in total serum cholesterol were explained by differences in daily caloric intake."

The other neat piece of information that you can determine with this percentage is the amount of the differences in total serum cholesterol that were related to factors other than daily caloric intake (e.g., genetics, exercise, etc.). That amount is the difference between the percentage of variance and 100%, in this case, $100\% - 49\% = 51\%$. In terms of clinical importance, any value of $r > 0.3$ (which you know means that it explains about 9% of the variance) is considered clinically important (Grove, 2007). Now that is pretty understandable!

You can also use the Pearson's correlation coefficient (r) to determine the effect size to use when calculating sample size. Think about it: The effect size is just an estimate of the relationship/difference you are attempting to find.

- When you have a strong correlation, you have a large effect size and don't need such a large sample to find a statistically significant difference if it exists.
- When the strength of the correlation is weak, the effect size is small, and you need a larger sample to detect statistically significant differences.

For example, when Pearson's $r = 0.4$, one of your variables explains 16% of the variance in the other, which is considered a medium effect size. When Pearson's $r = 0.6$, one of your variables explains 36% of the variance of the other, which is a large effect size. You will need a larger sample to detect the small or medium correlation (i.e., $r = 0.4$) and a smaller sample when you are trying to detect the large correlation (i.e., $r = 0.6$). (I told you it made sense.)

FROM THE STATISTICIAN *Brendan Heavey*

Methods: Correlation Coefficients

Here is an example of how to use correlation coefficients. The director of the local community center believes that students are at increased risk for accidental injury as they progress through the higher grades in high school. He wants to know how these two variables (increased risk of accidental injury and grade level) are related in the population that the center serves. He gives you a database with randomly collected surveys of 108 adolescents who participate at the center and asks you to complete an analysis. You note two questions in particular: One asks the students to identify their current grade, and another asks how often the students experienced an accidental injury in the last 6 months. Injury risk is coded 1–5: 1 = never, 2 = less than three times, 3 = three to five times, 4 = five to seven times, 5 = more than seven times. You decide to analyze these two variables using a correlation coefficient. Being the statistical genius that you are, you know that identifying the correct correlation coefficient for the job means answering a few questions.

First, do you have one independent sample? In this example, the data you have was collected from adolescents at one community center. There is no contrasting sample, and you are not dividing the sample into different samples to compare. Each of the adolescents was surveyed only once, and they are not related in any way. Therefore, you have one independent sample.

Second, you need to be sure that you are looking for a linear relationship between two variables, and you are.

Last, you must identify the level of measurement of the variables in order to select the correct correlation coefficient. The first variable is the current grade level of the student, which is interval/ratio level. The level of measurement of injury risk is ordinal (the intervals are not equal, so don't be misled by the coding).

You can now identify which correlation coefficient is appropriate for this sample. Your statistical program outputs the tables shown in **Tables 11-1** and **11-2**. Which table is appropriate for your analysis, and why?

TABLE 11-1	**Correlation Coefficient: Table 1**

Correlations

			Risk	Grade
Pearson's *r*	Risk	Pearson's correlation	1.000	0.159
		Significance (two-tailed)		0.101
		N	108.000	108
	Grade	Pearson correlation	0.159	1.000
		Significance (two-tailed)	0.101	
		N	108	108.000

(continues)

FROM THE STATISTICIAN *Brendan Heavey*

TABLE 11-2	**Correlation Coefficient: Table 2**			
			Risk	**Grade**
Spearman's ρ	Risk	Correlation coefficient	1.000	0.156
		Significance (two-tailed)		0.106
		N	108	108
	Grade	Correlation coefficient	0.156	1.000
		Significance (two-tailed)	0.106	
		N	108	108

Because you know your risk variable is ordinal, you know you must use the Spearman ρ correlation coefficient in Table 11-2. (If it were interval or ratio, you could use Table 11-1 and the Pearson's correlation coefficient.) Looking at Table 11-2, you can determine that the correlation between the risk of injury and the student's grade level is actually 0.156. Of course, you also know that the p-value associated with this correlation is 0.106, which is not significant. You are then able to report to the community center director that, unfortunately, the grade level explains only 2.4% (0.156 $\times$ 0.156) of the variance in accidental injury in this sample. It is not significantly related to the risk for accidental injury.

Before you wrap up this analysis, go back to Table 11-2 and make sure you understand what the other numbers mean. Don't worry—they're pretty straightforward. First, you know that $N = 108$ means that 108 adolescents were in your sample. But why is 1.00 listed as the correlation coefficient between grade and grade and between risk and risk? That number shows that when you correlate a variable with itself, the correlation coefficient is 1.00. It is a perfect correlation. Any variable should correlate perfectly with itself!

SUMMARY

Good job completing the chapter! Now we will review the concepts.

A correlation is the relationship between two variables.

- You use the chi-square test to look for a correlation when you have an independent sample and the variables are both categorical (nominal or ordinal).

- The Spearman correlation coefficient is used if the variable examined are ordinal, interval, or ratio level and don't meet the Pearson's assumptions, such as normality of distribution.
- If you have two normally distributed interval- or ratio-level variables, the Pearson's correlation coefficient is used.

Both the Spearman and Pearson's correlation coefficients tell you the direction and strength of the linear relationship between the two variables. The direction of the relationship can be either positive or negative. In a positive correlation, as one variable increases, so does the other; as one variable decreases, so does the other. In a negative correlation, as one variable increases, the second variable decreases; as one variable decreases, the second increases.

The strength of the relationship is determined by the absolute value of the correlation coefficient. The coefficient of determination is represented by r^2 because you must square Pearson's r. The percentage of variance is the amount of variance in one variable that is explained by the second variable, and it is determined by multiplying the coefficient of determination (r^2) by 100.

These concepts may be a little confusing, so review this chapter until you feel completely confident. Keep your head up, and continue to study hard. Believe it or not, the concepts eventually sink in as you continue to use them. Do you remember learning how to take a blood pressure? I thought I'd never master the skill, and I felt very, very anxious. Now blood pressures are old hat. Statistics is the same; you just need to practice until the concepts make sense. The more you use them, the clearer they become.

THINKING IT THROUGH

Correlation of Variables

Tests that look for an association between variables in **one group or sample (no comparison group)**:*

Variables Involved in the Association Being Tested	Test	Example
Nominal/ordinal	Chi-square	Is there an association between shift worked and marital status among nurses at my hospital?
Ordinal and Ordinal **Ordinal and Interval/ratio (if not normally distributed)**	Spearman's correlation	Is there an association between heart rate (HR) and pain in hospitalized children? (HR measured as beats per minute; pain measured as mild/moderate/severe.)
Interval/ratio	Pearson's correlation	Is there an association between heart rate and blood pressure among men attending an Alcoholics Anonymous meeting?

* These tests simply look for associations or relationships, not differences between groups. For example, in a sample of nurses working extended shifts, a relationship was found between hours worked and the number of medication errors.

CHAPTER 11 REVIEW QUESTIONS

Questions 1–18: You are asked to conduct a study to determine whether there is an association between consumption of milk proteins and levels of serum antibodies in children with autism. You randomly select 50 children previously enrolled in an autism clinical trial, and they are the sample for the study. You select an alpha of 0.05 and a power of 0.80.

1. Your study measures consumption of milk proteins as a yes/no question. It measures serum antibodies as a present/not present question. What level are the two variables?

2. What analysis method do you propose based on this information?

3. Your research partner believes it would be better to measure milk protein consumption as a low/moderate/high question and to quantify the serum antibody level by using the actual amount present. If you take this approach, what analysis method do you propose?

4. The biostatistician in your department recommends that you change your milk protein measurement to one that is the number of servings per day. You continue to use the actual quantity of the serum antibodies. What analysis method do you recommend?

5. Write an appropriate null hypothesis for this study.

6. Write an appropriate alternative hypothesis for this study.

7. Is your sample size large enough to conduct a correlation test? Is it large enough to assume a normal distribution and homoscedasticity?

8. You decide to utilize the measurement variables as recommended by the biostatistician and conduct a Pearson's correlation coefficient test. You determine $r = 0.6$. What must your p-value be for this to be statistically significant?

9. Your p-value is 0.08. Is this significant?

10. What do you conclude?

11. Suppose that you were able to refine your measurement tools and repeat the study. This time you determine you had an r of 0.6 with a p-value of 0.049. What would you conclude?

12. This information would let you know that your original conclusion was actually what type of error?

13. What is the strength of the relationship between consumption of milk proteins and serum antibodies?

14. Is the relationship positive or negative? Interpret this in plain English.

15. In this study, what percentage of variance in serum antibody levels is explained by the consumption of milk proteins in children with autism?

16. How much of the variance is explained by other variables?

17. Is this clinically important?

18. If you were going to use this effect size to determine your sample size for another study, would you expect to need a large or a small sample?

Questions 19–24: You develop a screening test to be used for children with autism to detect serum antibodies from milk protein consumption and have the following 2 × 2 table.

	Disease	**No Disease**	**Totals**
Positive test	10	2	12
Negative test	3	220	223
Totals	13	222	235

Calculate the following values:

19. Sensitivity:

20. Specificity:

21. Positive predictive value:

22. Negative predictive value:

23. Prevalence:

24. If early treatment helps, is this a good screen?

Questions 25–27: You are asked to complete a study for a small school district that is trying to keep as many students at age-appropriate grade levels as possible. You have a measure of grade level and age for the students, as well as the following statistical programming output from a randomized independent sample:

Correlations

			Age	Grade
Pearson's *r*	Age	Pearson correlation	1.000	0.382*
		Significance (two-tailed)		0.000
		N	108.000	108
	Grade	Pearson correlation	0.382*	1.000
		Significance (two-tailed)	0.000	
		N	108	108.000

* Correlation is significant at the 0.01 level (two-tailed).

Correlations

			Age	Grade
Spearman's *ρ*	Age	Correlation coefficient	1.000	0.378*
		Significance (two-tailed)		0.000
		N	108	108
	Grade	Correlation coefficient	0.378	1.000
		Significance (two-tailed)	0.000	
		N	108	108

* Correlation is significant at the 0.01 level (two-tailed).

25. What is your sample size?

26. What is the appropriate correlation coefficient, and why?

27. Are age and grade significantly correlated?

Questions 28–30: A nurse researcher conducts a study to determine if taking a new fertility drug is associated with multiple-fetus pregnancies. Her sample includes 500 women who are pregnant in her fertility practice. She selects an alpha of 0.05 and a power of 0.80.

28. If taking the new drug is measured as yes/no, what level of measurement is it?

29. If a multiple-fetus pregnancy is also measured as yes/no, what correlation test is appropriate, and why?

30. The researcher reports that $p = 0.044$. What conclusion should the researcher make about the null hypothesis? Why?

Question 31–39: A researcher conducts a study to determine if there is an association between time spent in solitary confinement and depression rates in 120 male prisoners. The alpha is 0.05, and the power is 0.80.

31. If time spent in solitary confinement is measured in total hours, what level of measurement is this variable?

32. If depression is measured on a scale with values from 1 to 10, what level of measurement is the variable?

33. What would be the appropriate correlation test, and why?

34. The study reports that $r = 0.4$. What does this mean in plain English?

35. How much of the variance in depression is explained by hours in solitary confinement?

36. If $p = 0.07$, is the correlation significant? Why or why not?

37. If the hypothesis decision is incorrect, what type of error could it be?

38. If instead the study measured time in solitary confinement as none, infrequent, or regular, what level of measurement would it be?

39. Would this change the correlation test you would recommend? Why or why not?

Research Application Article

Look at the following research article to see how the statistical techniques you have already learned are used in practice:

Watson, J., Kinstler, A., Vidonish III, W. P., Wagner, M., Li, L., Davis, K. G., . . . Daraiseh, N. M. (2015). Impact of noise on nurses in pediatric intensive care units. *American Journal of Critical Care, 24*(5), 377–384. doi:10.4037/ajcc2015260

1. What was the purpose of this study?
2. What type of sample was collected?
3. What are the noise-level recommendations from the Environmental Protection Agency (EPA) and the World Health Organization (WHO)?
4. Why does the noise level in the workplace matter?
5. The sample included nurses from what units?
6. What nurses from these units were not included in the study?
7. How was noise level measured? What level of measurement is this variable?
8. How was heart rate measured? What level of measurement is this variable?
9. How was stress measured? What level of measurement is this variable?
10. In addition to the noise-level measurement, the observer log recorded what information about the noise? What level of measurement was this additional information?
11. Look at Table 2 in the article. Which unit, on average, was the loudest?
12. Look at Table 2 in the article. Which unit was the quietest on average? Was this unit within the recommended EPA guidelines for workplace sound levels?
13. Look at Table 2 in the article. What percentage of the time was the noise level of the Cardiac Intensive Care Unit (CICU) over the cutoff level that the National Institute on Deafness and Other Communication Disorders (NIDOCD) indicated can cause physiological damage?
14. If you were a nurse working in the CICU, would this finding concern you?
15. What does this study tell you about the noise level on the weekend? Based on this study, would you be more or less concerned about noise levels on the weekend?
16. Look at Table 2 in the article. Which location on the units was the noisiest on average (sound pressure level [SPL]? How noisy was it on average?
17. Look at Table 2 in the article. Were patient interactions or employee interactions louder?
18. The sample was found to reflect the same gender and age distribution of the population of inpatient nurses within this facility. What does this mean about the representativeness of the sample for this facility? Of a national population of nurses from all inpatient facilities? How does this affect the generalizability of the study results?
19. In the statistical analysis and results section, the authors report that the noise level in the three units was compared. Because they were comparing three groups, what statistical test was utilized, and where were significant differences found? The researchers later offer an explanation for why this may be the case. What explanation is provided?
20. Look at Table 3 in the article. What was the most frequent source of noise?
21. Look at Table 3 in the article. What was the most frequent location of noise?
22. Look at Table 3 in the article. What was the most frequent source of noise that was $>$ 75 dBA?
23. Look at Table 5 in the article. Pearson correlation coefficients were calculated to determine the association between heart rate and noise level (SPL). What do you know about the overall correlation between these two variables in this sample?
24. Calculate the coefficient of determination. What percentage of variance in heart rate is explained by the noise level in the overall relationship?
25. Look at Table 5 in the article. Was this correlation between heart rate and noise level (SPL) seen in the CICU?

26. Look at Table 5 in the article. At what noise location is the correlation between heart rate and noise level the strongest?
27. The researchers indicate that significant positive correlations were found between heart rate and noise levels in patients' rooms, communicating with staff and between patients and their families and during all nursing activities. They explain that direct care may be a confounding factor for this finding. Explain what this means in your own words.

ANSWERS TO ODD-NUMBERED CHAPTER 11 REVIEW QUESTIONS

1. Both nominal

3. Ordinal/ratio—Spearman's correlation coefficient

5. H_0: There is no association between milk protein consumption and serum antibodies.

7. Yes, it is greater than or equal to 3; yes, it is greater than or equal to 50.

9. No

11. Reject the null; there is a relationship.

13. $0.6 =$ strong

15. $0.6 \times 0.6 = 0.36 = 36\%$

17. Yes, $> 9\%$

19. $10 \div 13 = 0.77$, or 77%

21. $10 \div 12 = 0.83$, or 83%

23. $13 \div 235 = 0.06$, or 6%

25. 108 students

27. $r = 0.382$, which is significant ($p < 0.01$).

29. Chi-square, both nominal level

31. Ratio

33. Pearson's—both are interval/ratio, and sample > 50.

35. $r^2 \times 100 = 0.16 \times 100 = 16\%$

37. Type two

39. Yes. The ordinal variable means you would need to do a Spearman's correlation now.

Research Application Article

1. To determine if there is an association between noise levels and health in a sample of nurses
3. Sound pressure levels (SPLs) in hospitals should be less than 45 dBA during the day and 35 dBA during the night. The World Health Organization recommends an 8-hour weight average of <30 dBA with peaks <40 dBA.
5. NICU, CICU, and PICU
7. Noise level was measured with a noise dosimeter in SPLs in decibels at 1-minute intervals. This is a ratio level of measurement.
9. Stress was measured using the Specific Rating of Events Scale (0–100) at the beginning of, at the midpoint, and after the observation. This is a ratio level of measurement that was repeated.
11. The CICU (mean $= 73.8$ dBA).
13. NIDOCD indicates that levels >75 dBA can cause physiological damage. The CICU had noise levels over this level 39.5% of the time.
15. Nothing. The noise levels were recorded only Monday through Friday. You are unable to determine if you would be more or less concerned about noise levels on the weekend.
17. Employee interactions (mean $= 73.4$ dBA) were louder than patient interactions (mean $= 69.6$ dBA).

19. The researchers conducted an ANOVA test and report significantly higher noise levels in the CICU versus the PICU ($p < 0.001$) and in the NICU versus the PICU ($p < 0.001$). The PICU was recently remodeled to include laminate plank flooring, which is noted to reduce noise. The flooring in the CICU and the NICU were vinyl composite tile.

21. Patients' rooms

23. There is a significant but weak, positive correlation between heart rate and noise level (SPL) ($r = 0.19, p < 0.001$).

25. No. In the CICU, the researchers report a nonsignificant, very weak, negative correlation between the variables ($r = -0.03, p = 0.71$).

27. Answers will vary. For example: A confounding factor is related to both study variables, making it more challenging to determine the actual relationship between the two variables without controlling for the confounding factor. In this example, the significantly positive correlation between noise and heart rate may mean that there is more noise when providing direct patient care and that heart rate goes up while providing direct patient care. Once the role of direct patient care is controlled (for example, looking at the relationship between noise and heart rate only among nurses providing direct patient care), the researchers may not find a significant relationship between the noise level and heart rate.

CHAPTER 12

REGRESSION ANALYSIS

QUANTIFYING AN ASSOCIATION
TO PREDICT FUTURE EVENTS

OBJECTIVES

By the end of this chapter students will be able to:

- Identify the conditions under which regression is an appropriate statistical technique.

- Compare and contrast linear regression, multiple regression, and logistic regression.

- Explain how quantifying an association with a regression equation helps a researcher infer or predict future events.

- Use regression coefficients to interpret how a change in the independent variable affects the predicted value of the dependent variable.

- Contrast positive and negative regression coefficients.

- Discuss when reporting an adjusted R-squared is more appropriate.

- Interpret the Statistical Package for the Social Sciences (SPSS) output utilizing multiple regression, determine whether the model as well as the independent variables are significant, and interpret these results in statistical terms and in plain English.

- Critique an article from current nursing research that utilizes a regression technique, determine whether statistical significance is present, and debate whether clinical recommendations should be made.

KEY TERMS

Adjusted *R*-squared

Value reported to avoid overestimating the percentage of variance in the outcome explained by the model, such as when there are a large number of independent variables with a relatively small sample size.

Linear regression

Technique for analyzing the relationship between a single independent variable and a single interval- or ratio-level dependent variable, enabling the researcher to make a prediction about a future outcome based on the research data included in the analysis.

Logistic regression

Method for analyzing the relationship between multiple independent variables and a single dependent or outcome variable when the outcome is binary (has only two categories).

Multiple regression

A statistical method used to look at the relationship between a dependent variable and multiple independent variables to develop a prediction equation based on the research data included in the analysis.

Odds ratio (OR)

The odds or probability of the outcome occurring divided by the odds or probability of the outcome not occurring.

R-squared change

The change in the percentage of the variance in the outcome variable (R^2) that is explained by the model with the addition of another independent variable.

R-squared value (R^2)

The percentage of the variance in the dependent or outcome variable that is explained by the model.

Regression

A statistical technique that allows the researcher to make a prediction about a future outcome based on the research data included.

Regression coefficient

The b value, which tells you the rate of change in the outcome or dependent variable with a one-unit increase in the corresponding independent variable.

Residual

The amount of prediction error in a regression equation.

Standard error of the estimate

The average amount of error there will be in the predicted outcome using a model.

QUANTIFYING AN ASSOCIATION

It is one thing to recognize statistically significant relationships and another to be able to use that information to begin the process of inferring or predicting future events. In order to do that, we first need to quantify the association. Let's look at an example. Most obstetric nurses have read the literature showing a significant relationship between smoking and fetal weight. This is helpful knowledge to have for our pregnant patients. However, if you have a patient who is smoking 10 cigarettes a day and really doesn't want to quit, she may not think smoking 10 cigarettes a day will have that much of an impact on the size of her baby. Just being able to tell her there is a statistically significant correlation between smoking and fetal weight may not be enough.

You are going to need to use more statistics before you can convince this patient that it is important for her to quit smoking.

You know that correlations measure the strength of associations; now we want to be able to quantify that association, which involves one of my favorite statistical techniques, called **regression**. No, we are not all going to take a moment and relive childhood memories. This is math, remember, but it can still be fun! Regression happens to be a favorite test of mine for one basic reason—developing an accurate regression equation is the first step in being able to predict future events. It is like being a psychic—but this time your predictions should actually be true!

Of course, there isn't just one kind of regression analysis, so let's start with the most basic, although not one that is used that often in the literature. You need to understand the basics of **linear regression** before you understand the more complex types of regression, so it is a good place to begin.

Linear regression looks for a relationship between a single independent variable and a single interval- or ratio-level dependent variable. (You can sometimes use this technique when you have ordinal-level dependent variables as well, but it gets a little more complicated.) Once the temporality of the relationship is established, you can then make an inference or a prediction about the future value of the dependent variable at a given level of the independent variable. In the fetal weight example, you might use linear regression to see the relationship between the number of cigarettes smoked each day and fetal weight. Maybe knowing, for example, that for every five cigarettes a day a patient doesn't smoke, her baby will weigh about a half a pound more will help motivate your pregnant patient to decrease her cigarette smoking.

FROM THE STATISTICIAN *Brendan Heavey*

Statistics, Jerry Springer Style: Now Let's Look at Some Relationships That Aren't Functional!

Regression is a method that allows us to examine the relationship between two or more variables. You may recall another way of exploring the relationship between two variables from earlier in life when you first learned to graph the formula of a line using the formula $Y = mX + b$. Remember what all these letters represent:

Y is the dependent variable and is displayed on the vertical axis.
X is the independent variable and is displayed on the horizontal axis.
M is the slope and represents the amount of change in the Y variable for each unit change in the X variable.
b is the Y-intercept, and it tells us the value of Y when the line crosses the vertical axis ($X = 0$).

In this relationship, the value of the variable Y varies according to the value of X based on the values of two constants, or parameters. If you know the values of m, X, and b, you can solve for the value of Y exactly. Let's look at

(continues)

FROM THE STATISTICIAN *Brendan Heavey*

an example. In the graph shown in **Figure 12-1**, you can see three functional relationships between the total cost of three different types of treatment for minor wound infections in June. Treatment 1, outpatient treatment, is cheaper per unit, so there is a more gradual rise in overall cost for each additional treated case. Because all three treatments pass through the origin, their Y-intercepts are all 0. In fact, the only differences between these three lines are their slopes. Their equations are:

Treatment 1 (outpatient)—$250/case: $Y = 250\,X$
Treatment 2 (inpatient medical treatment)—$500/case: $Y = 500\,X$
Treatment 3 (same-day surgical treatment)—$750/case: $Y = 750\,X$

This math is all well and good, but things rarely work out this nicely in nature. The problem that usually occurs is that the relationship between most variables, just like the relationship between many people, is not functional. Can you guess what term best describes the relationship between almost all variables? Why, *statistical*, of course! You see, the difference between a functional relationship and a statistical relationship is that a statistical relationship accounts for error.

FIGURE 12-1   **Relationship between Total Cost and Number of Patients Treated (Functional Relationship).**

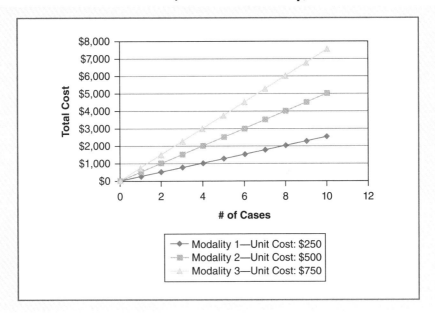

FROM THE STATISTICIAN *Brendan Heavey*

As it turns out, accounting for error is a very difficult task. We rarely, if ever, know how error is distributed around a mean value, so we usually have to make a few assumptions to allow us to make sense of our data.

In this text, we are doing our best to keep things simple and give you a basic introduction to regression, so we will stick with one of the most basic regression models available, namely, the *normal error regression model.* In this model, our most basic assumption is that the error we model is normally distributed around the mean of *Y.* This is okay to do, especially as our sample size is increased. Do you remember why? It is because of the central limit theorem. Because the distribution of the sum of random variables approaches normal as the number of variables is increased, and as our sample size increases, the amount of random error increases, we can assume that the distribution of this random error approaches normality. It is okay to make this assumption as long as you have a large enough sample. It is important to note that a few other assumptions are used in the normal error regression model, but they are beyond the scope of this text and most aspects of life.

So now let's look at what a statistical relationship or *statistical model* looks like. Here is the definition of the normal error regression model:

$$Y_i = \beta_0 + \beta_1 X_i + \varepsilon_i$$

In this model, there are three variables and two parameters (one more than the functional model you just saw). Here is what each of these terms means:

Y_i: The value of the dependent variable in the *i*th observation
X_i: The value of the independent variable in the *i*th observation
ε_i: The normally distributed error variable
β_0 and β_1 are parameters, just like the slope, *m*, and the *Y*-intercept (*b*) were in the functional relationship earlier.

Let's say we now have a little more information on treatment 1 (outpatient management) from our previous example. In this case, although there was an exact functional relationship between number of cases and total cost, when we look at the relationship between unit cost and time, it looks like this:

Cost of Treatment 1 throughout the Year

January	$118
February	$150
March	$165
April	$205
May	$215
June	$253

(continues)

FROM THE STATISTICIAN *Brendan Heavey*

Cost of Treatment 1 throughout the Year
(*Continued*)

July	$276
August	$289
September	$310
October	$325
November	$332
December	$362
Average	$250

There is not an exact functional relationship. In fact, the unit cost is increasing over time, but the amount of each increase is different each month. The increase in cost per month varies according to a few different factors, but you can see that if we graph this data, the trendline shows that unit cost is increasing, on average, $21.72 per month (see **Figure 12-2**).

FIGURE 12-2   **Unit Cost by Month for Treatment 1.**

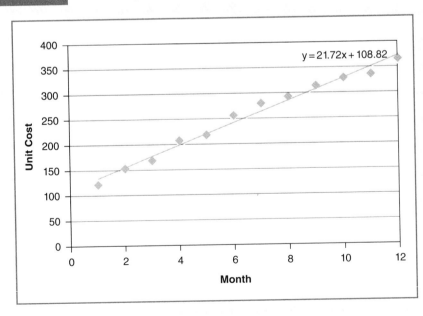

$y = 21.72x + 108.82$

FROM THE STATISTICIAN *Brendan Heavey*

Notice that you can see the error in this relationship. The trendline shows you a functional relationship that is buried inside the statistical relationship. The functional relationship is exactly quantified by two parameters and two variables:

$$Y = 21.72X + 108.82$$

The statistical relationship adds a third variable (error, ε), which allows the points on the graph the freedom to vary around this functional relationship because statistical relationships are never exact:

$$Y = 21.72X + 108.82 + \varepsilon$$

FIGURE 12-3   **Fetal Weight at Various Levels of Daily Cigarette Consumption.**

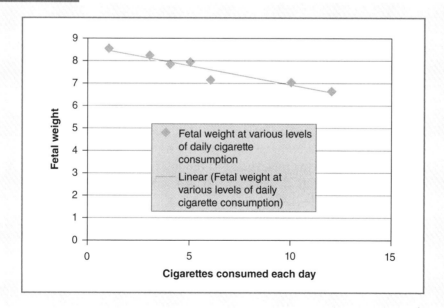

Linear regression plots out the values of the dependent variable (i.e., fetal weight) on the y-axis and the values of the independent variable (i.e., daily number of cigarettes) on the x-axis to find the line to illustrate the relationship between the two variables best (see **Figure 12-3**).

Assuming there is a linear relationship (you can see how a trendline is not exactly on the points of data, but the points follow it pretty closely or in a linear fashion), this line can then be used to make predictions about the future value of the dependent variable at the different levels of the independent variable. The difference between where the points of data actually fall and where the line predicts they will fall is something called a **residual**, or the prediction error, which is discussed further in the next "From the Statistician: Methods" feature. The lower the amount of residual, the better the line fits the actual data points.

The slope of the trendline tells how much the predicted value of the dependent variable changes when there is a one-unit change in the independent variable. In our example, the slope of the line would tell us how much the predicted fetal weight would drop with the consumption of an additional cigarette each day. Seems simple enough, right?

Unfortunately, life is rarely so simple, and statistics has to keep up with it. (And you thought statistics was what made life complicated!) Very rarely is there only one independent variable we need to consider, which may leave you asking: What do you do when you want to predict how two or more variables will affect the dependent or outcome variable? For example, the length of the pregnancy as well as the number of cigarettes smoked each day both affect fetal weight. You would not want to predict fetal weight with just one of these independent variables; you would want to include both. How can you make an accurate prediction in this situation? (No, no,

don't use the crystal ball. . . .) You just need to use another statistical test called **multiple regression**.

So let's go back to the example of studying fetal weight. Multiple regression lets us take the data we have measuring months pregnant (independent variable number 1 or X_1) and the number of cigarettes smoked (independent variable number 2 or X_2) and see how these variables relate and affect the outcome, which is fetal weight (dependent variable or Y). Using this example, the relationship can be expressed in an equation like this:

$$Y_i = a + b_1 X_1 + b_2 X_2 + e$$

Now I know many of you just looked at this equation and started to think, what on earth does this equation mean? Don't panic. Let's break it apart.

Y_i is just the value of your dependent variable, in this case, how much the fetus weighs.

The value of a is what is called the constant, or the value of Y when the value of X is 0. In our example, this would be the value of Y or fetal weight when the patient is not yet 1 month pregnant and has not smoked any cigarettes. Obviously, there would still be some fetal weight, although in this example a is probably going to be a very small number.

b_1 is the value of the **regression coefficient** for our first independent variable. It is the rate of change in the outcome for every one-unit increase in the first independent variable. In our example, it is how much we would expect fetal weight to increase for each additional month of pregnancy.

What Is a Residual?

Consider the following data, which shows the results of a survey that collected IQ level on a series of patients with elevated blood lead levels (BLLs).

Obs.	BLL (mcg/dL)	IQ
1	7	125
2	18	109
3	22	110
4	25	117
5	29	110
6	37	98
7	44	94
8	56	90
9	64	84
10	100	81

Now, you can see in **Figure 12-4** what this data looks like when we graph it. Let's look at this model a little more in depth. To do so, we'll need two definitions:

- We refer to the fitted value of our regression function (or the inferred value of the dependent variable) at a particular X value as $\hat{Y}$ (pronounced Y-hat). Because the formula for our regression line is $\hat{Y} = -0.4886X + 121.4428$, if we are interested in the fitted value at an X of 7, we solve for $\hat{Y}$ like this:

$$\hat{Y} = -0.4886(7) + 121.4428$$

$$\hat{Y} = -3.4202 + 121.4428$$

$$= 118.0226$$

This means that at a blood lead level of 7, our regression model infers an IQ of 118.0226 on the y-axis.

- We refer to the distance between the actual observed value and the regression line as a *residual*, which is usually labeled using the Greek symbol **ε**. On a graph, it looks like **Figure 12-5**.

(continues)

FROM THE STATISTICIAN *Brendan Heavey*

FIGURE 12-4   **IQ versus BLL.**

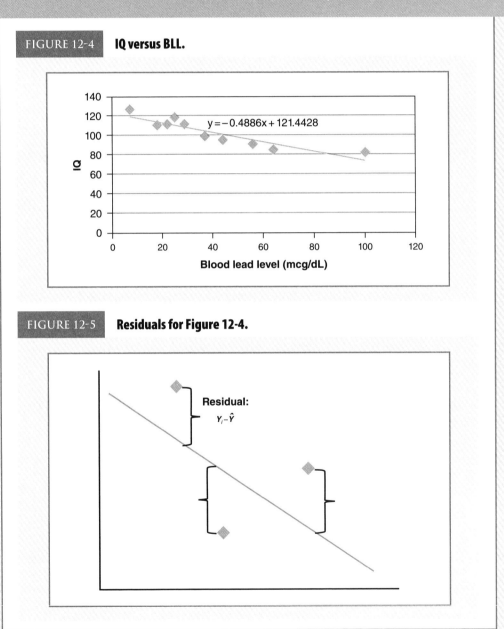

FIGURE 12-5   **Residuals for Figure 12-4.**

FROM THE STATISTICIAN *Brendan Heavey*

In this example, the fitted regression function equals 118.02 at an X of 7. Now, look at the data we observed to come up with this regression line. The observed value at an X of 7 was 125. Therefore, our residual value at an X of 7 is:

$$\varepsilon = 125 - 118.02 = 6.98$$

Let's look at the data from our example and calculate the residuals for our model. Plug in each of the X's to solve for $\hat{Y}$, and then subtract from the actual observed value to get the residual:

Observation	Blood Lead Level (mcg/dL)	IQ (Y_i)	$\hat{Y}$	Residual
1	7	125	118.02	6.98
2	18	109	112.65	3.65
3	22	110	110.69	0.69
4	25	117	109.23	7.77
5	29	110	107.27	2.73
6	37	98	103.36	5.36
7	44	94	99.94	5.94
8	56	90	94.08	4.08
9	64	84	90.17	6.17
10	100	81	72.58	8.32
			Sum	0

Notice that if you sum the residuals, you get a total of 0. This is always true for the normal error linear regression model.

Finally, it is important to point out the distinction between residuals and error. Remember the normal error regression model:

$$Y_i = \beta_0 + \beta_1 X_i + \varepsilon_i$$

It is really easy to confuse the final variable in this model, which represents the error, with residuals. Remember, residuals are a real construct. They are easily calculated from observed data. They represent observed error. The error term in the model is more abstract. It represents all error from the entire model, which has a much larger range than our observed data.

X_1 is the value of our first independent variable, or, in this example, how many months pregnant the patient is at the time of measurement.

b_2 is the value of the regression coefficient for the second independent variable. It is the rate of change in the outcome for every one-unit increase in the second independent variable. In our example, it is how much change we would expect in fetal weight when one additional cigarette is smoked every day. In all likelihood, the value of b_2 would be negative in this example because increases in daily cigarette consumption usually lower fetal weight. If the value of the regression coefficient is negative, an increase in the corresponding independent variable produces a decrease in the dependent or outcome variable, such as an increase in cigarette consumption producing a decrease in fetal weight.

Last, there is always an error term in statistics, and in this equation, it is represented by the e. Just as there are no perfect people, there are no perfect estimates. The e just acknowledges that these statistical procedures are estimates taken from a sample, not the parameters you would find in a population model.

So if we wanted to put the previous equation into plain English using our example, we would say:

Fetal weight $=$ a baseline value $+$ an amount related to the length of the pregnancy $+$ an amount related to the number of cigarettes smoked (probably negative) $+$ a certain amount of error

Now hopefully that makes a little more sense.

Once you put in the data you have about the duration of the pregnancy and the number of cigarettes smoked, assuming this is a good regression equation, you should be able to predict an accurate fetal weight. For example, after we compute the regression equation, we determine the following:

$$Y = 0.25 + 0.79X_1 - 0.15X_2 + 0.5$$

A patient comes into your unit who is having some preterm labor at 7.5 months. She reports smoking 10 cigarettes a day. You might be concerned because you would predict the current fetal weight to be only 5.18 pounds.

$$Y = 0.25 + 0.79(7.5) - 0.15(10) + 0.5$$

$$Y = 5.175 \text{ pounds}$$

Given that information, you might anticipate transferring the patient to a tertiary care facility if you are unable to stop the preterm labor.

Now the next question becomes: How do you know if you have a good regression equation? See, I knew you were going to ask that! Let's look at some computer output to answer that question. There is another piece of good news when it comes to regression analysis, which is that you are not going to do any of the calculations yourself. We are going to make the computer do all the hard work, and then we are going to look at the results and see what we have figured out. However, for those of you who like to see the math to help understand the concept, check out the "From the Statistician: Methods" feature, where you can learn to calculate the regression coefficients manually.

FROM THE STATISTICIAN *Brendan Heavey*

Calculating Regression Coefficients (Parameter Estimates)

Regression coefficients (parameter estimates) can be calculated in many ways; the method you probably will choose is to use some computer software package to spit them out. However, I think it is an important exercise to see just what that computer package is doing behind the scenes.

Remember, the normal error simple linear regression model we have been looking at thus far is:

$$Y_i = \beta_0 + \beta_1 X_i + \varepsilon_i$$

This model represents how variables and parameters interact in a population. The true values for the parameters β_1 and β_2 are never really known. However, when we sample real data from a population, we can come up with very good estimates of what these parameters are, given a few reasonable assumptions, by using the following two equations. Notice, we need the result of the first equation to solve the second equation:

$$b_1 = \frac{\sum (X_i - \overline{X})(Y_i - \overline{Y})}{\sum (X_i - \overline{X})^2}$$

$$b_0 = \overline{Y} - b_1 \overline{X}$$

These equations are called the *normal equations* and are derived using a process called *ordinary least squares*. To calculate these parameters, the first thing we do is find the denominator in the equation for b_1:

$$\sum (X_i - \overline{X})^2$$

This denominator is an example of a very important concept in statistics called a *sum of squares*, which is calculated by subtracting the mean of a set of values from each of the observed values, squaring it, and then summing the results over the whole set. For instance, if we have a data set with two values:

$$X = \{5, 15\}$$

Our mean value, $\overline{X} = 10$ and

$$\sum (X_i - \overline{X})^2 = (5 - 10)^2 + (15 - 10)^2$$
$$= -5^2 + 5^2$$
$$= 25 + 25$$

(continues)

FROM THE STATISTICIAN *Brendan Heavey*

Notice that a value that is 5 below the mean and a value that is 5 above the mean both get the same amount of weight included in the overall sum (25 each). This sum allows us to quantify the overall distance away from the mean value that our data set contains, whether that distance is positive or negative.

The concept of a sum of squares is important for a number of reasons, not the least of which is that the equations we use to solve for our regression parameters are derived by calculating all possible sums of squared error in our regression model and selecting the one with the minimum error (also known in calculus as minimizing the sum of squared error). We will revisit the concept of a sum of squares when we learn about multiple regression analysis later in this chapter. Now there is a cliffhanger for you!

For now, let's get back to solving for our estimates of the linear regression model by using data from our last "From the Statistician" feature, reproduced here:

Observation	Blood Lead Level (mcg/dL)	IQ (Y_i)
1	7	125
2	18	109
3	22	110
4	25	117
5	29	110
6	37	98
7	44	94
8	56	90
9	64	84
10	100	81

You can see from our formulas that in order to solve for b_1, we need to solve for $\overline{X}$ before we can solve for the sum of squares in the denominator. To do this, simply take the average of all our X's:

$$\overline{X} = \frac{7 + 18 + 22 + 25 + 29 + 37 + 44 + 56 + 64 + 100}{10}$$

$$= \frac{402}{10}$$

$$= 40.2$$

FROM THE STATISTICIAN *Brendan Heavey*

We now know that in our sample, the average BLL of the subjects is 40.2 mcg/dL. Now take each individual BLL (X) and subtract the mean BLL $\overline{X}$ we calculated for the whole sample and square the result (shown here in the third column):

X_i	$X_i - \overline{X}$	$(X_i - \overline{X})^2$
7	−33.2	1102.24
18	−22.2	492.84
22	−18.2	331.24
25	−15.2	231.04
29	−11.2	125.44
37	−3.2	10.24
44	3.8	14.44
56	15.8	249.64
64	23.8	566.44
100	59.8	3576.04

Now, sum the results of $(X_i - \overline{X})^2$:

$$\sum (X_i - \overline{X})^2 = 1102.25 + 492.84 + 331.24 + 231.04 + 125.44 + 10.24 + 14.44 + 249.64 + 566.44 + 3576.04$$

$$= 6699.6$$

The denominator of our first parameter, b_1, is 6699.6.

Now let's go back and find the numerator of b_1. First solve for the mean value of Y ($\overline{Y}$). To do so, simply add all the observed IQ values (Y) and divide by the number of observations, 10:

$$\overline{Y} = \frac{125 + 109 + 110 + 117 + 110 + 98 + 94 + 90 + 84 + 81}{10}$$

$$\overline{Y} = 101.8$$

(continues)

FROM THE STATISTICIAN   *Brendan Heavey*

Now, subtract $\overline{X}$ from each of the X's and $\overline{Y}$ from each of the Y's:

X_i	$X_i - \overline{X}$	Y_i	$Y_i - \overline{Y}$
7	−33.2	125	23.2
18	−22.2	109	7.2
22	−18.2	110	8.2
25	−15.2	117	15.2
29	−11.2	110	8.2
37	−3.2	98	−3.8
44	3.8	94	−7.8
56	15.8	90	−11.8
64	23.8	84	−17.8
100	59.8	81	−20.8

Now, multiply column 2 by column 4 in the above table and sum the result to get the numerator:

$X_i - \overline{X}$	$Y_i - \overline{Y}$	$(X_i - \overline{X}) * (Y_i - \overline{Y})$
−33.2	23.2	−770.24
−22.2	7.2	−159.84
−18.2	8.2	−149.24
−15.2	15.2	−231.04
−11.2	8.2	−91.84
−3.2	−3.8	12.16
3.8	−7.8	−29.64
15.8	−11.8	−186.44
23.8	−17.8	−423.64
59.8	−20.8	−1243.84
		−3273.6

FROM THE STATISTICIAN *Brendan Heavey*

Now, take this numerator, −3273.6, and divide by the denominator we solved for before, 6699.6:

$$b_i = \frac{\sum(X_i - \overline{X})(Y_i - \overline{Y})}{\sum(X_i - \overline{X})^2}$$

To come up with our first parameter estimate:

$$b_i = -0.48863$$

Now, because we know b_1, $\overline{Y}$, and $\overline{X}$, we can solve for b_0 pretty easily:

$$b_0 = \overline{Y} - b_0\overline{X}$$

$$= 101.8 - (-0.48862 * 40.2)$$

$$= 101.8 + 19.6429$$

$$= 121.4429$$

And now we have our regression equation:

$$Y_i = 121.4429 - 0.4886X_i$$

Notice we left out the error term. Do you remember how to calculate the error of the sampled values? The residuals! The residuals represent the distance between our observed values and our calculated regression line. However, because our residuals sum to 0, we can leave that term out when looking at our overall model.

Let's say I am interested in predicting an individual's weight. My study includes information about age and height. When I put that information into the computer and complete a regression analysis, I have the following output:

		Model Summary		
Model	**R**	**R-Squared**	**Adjusted R-Squared**	**Std. Error of the Estimate**
1	0.656[a]	0.430	0.367	31.24864
2	0.922[b]	0.850	0.813	16.99823

[a]Predictors: (Constant), age
[b]Predictors: (Constant), age, height

Let's look at each of these columns and figure out what the information means.

The first row (model 1) is when we only include the independent variable of age in the regression equation. The second row (model 2) is when we include age and then add the second independent variable of height to the model.

R is the multiple correlation coefficient that, when squared, gives you the **R-squared (R^2) value**. Great, you say, and what does that mean?

Well, R^2 is important because it tells you the percentage of the variance in the dependent or outcome variable that is explained by the model you have built. In this example, the R^2 of 0.850 on line 2 is when both age (independent variable one) and height (independent variable two) are included in the model. This just means including both age and height explains 85% of the variance seen in weight. See, not so bad. That R^2 is handy!

FROM THE STATISTICIAN *Brendan Heavey*

A Closer Look at *R*-Squared

R-squared is a fantastic tool and is often the single statistic used to determine whether we can use a particular regression model. To derive *R*-squared requires looking at a regression equation from a slightly different view. The output from most statistical packages will show us a table with this view of our model, namely, the analysis of variance or ANOVA table. It doesn't matter which package you choose to use; you will get almost all the same information on this table. Here's what the output looks like for the model in our previous example:

ANOVA[a]

Model	Sum of Squares	df	Mean Square	F	Sig.
1 Regression	1599.567	1	1599.567	39.985	0.000[b]
Residual	320.033	8	40.004		
Total	1919.600	9			

[a]Dependent variable: IQ
[b]Predictors: (Constant), BLL

Coefficients[a]

Model	Unstandardized Coefficients		Standardized Coefficients			
	B	Std. Error	Beta	t	Sig.	
1 (constant)	121.433	3.695	0.913	32.870	0.000	
BLL	−0.489	0.077		−6.323	0.000	

[a]Dependent variable: IQ

FROM THE STATISTICIAN *Brendan Heavey*

The three biggest concepts represented in the first table are:

- Sum of squares due to regression (SSR)
- Sum of squares due to error (labeled "Residual" here) (SSE)
- Total sum of squares

All three represent different reasons why *Y* values vary around their mean. Check out the diagram shown in **Figure 12-6**, which shows total deviation partitioned into two components, SSR and SSE, for the first observed value.

Here you can see how the total deviation of each observed *Y* value can be partitioned into two parts: the deviation due to the difference between the mean of *Y* and the regression line and the deviation between the observed value and the regression line. As it turns out, *R*-squared is simply the ratio of the second sum of squares over the total sum of squares.

| FIGURE 12-6 | **Partitioning the Total Deviation around $\overline{Y}$.** |

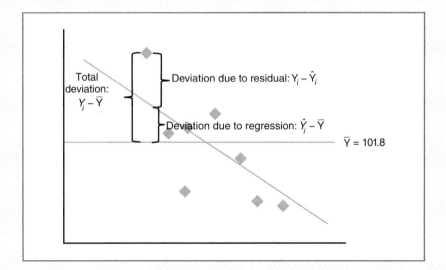

(continues)

FROM THE STATISTICIAN *Brendan Heavey*

Some variance is due to the regression itself, and some is due to error in the model. Here are the definitions of the sums of squares we're interested in, the total sum of squares (SST0), the sum of squares due to regression (SSR), and the sum of squares due to error (SSE).

1. $SST0 = \sum(Y_i - \overline{Y})^2$

SST0 represents the sum of the squared distance of each observed Y value from the overall mean of Y. You can see the distances that are squared and summed in Figure 12-6 under the heading "Total Deviation."

2. $SSR = \sum(\hat{Y}_i - \overline{Y})^2$

SSR represents the sum of the squared distance of the fitted regression line to the overall mean of Y. This is the variation that is due to the regression model itself.

3. $SSE = \sum(Y_i - \hat{Y}_i)^2$

SSE represents the sum of the squared distance between the observed Y values and the regression line. This is the variation that is due to difference between our observed values and our model, also known as the error in our model.

Let's take a minute and calculate these values by hand for the model in our example.

To calculate SST0, subtract each observed Y from the mean of Y, and square that value like this:

SST0			
IQ [Y_i]	$\overline{Y}$	$Y_i - \overline{Y}$	$(Y_i - \overline{Y})^2$
125	101.8	23.20	538.24
109	101.8	7.20	51.84
110	101.8	8.20	67.24
117	101.8	15.20	231.04
110	101.8	8.20	67.24
98	101.8	−3.80	14.44
94	101.8	−7.80	60.84
90	101.8	−11.80	139.24
84	101.8	−17.80	316.84
81	101.8	−20.80	432.64

FROM THE STATISTICIAN *Brendan Heavey*

Now, sum the right-most column, and we get our SST0:

$$SST0 = \sum (Y_i - \overline{Y})^2 = 1919.6$$

To calculate SSR, subtract the mean of Y from the fitted value on our regression line and square it:

SSR

$\hat{Y}$	$\overline{Y}$	$(\hat{Y} - \overline{Y})$	$(\hat{Y} - \overline{Y})^2$
118.02	101.8	16.22	263.17
112.65	101.8	10.85	117.67
110.69	101.8	8.89	79.09
109.23	101.8	7.43	55.16
107.27	101.8	5.47	29.95
103.36	101.8	1.56	2.44
99.94	101.8	−1.86	3.45
94.08	101.8	−7.72	59.60
90.17	101.8	−11.63	135.24
72.58	101.8	−29.22	853.80

Now, sum the right-most column, and we come up with the SSR:

$$SSR = \sum (\hat{Y} - \overline{Y})^2 = 1599.57$$

To calculate SSE, subtract the value of the regression line from each observed Y value and square it, like this:

SSE

IQ $[Y_i]$	$\hat{Y}$	$(Y_i - \hat{Y}_i)$	$(Y_i - \hat{Y}_i)^2$
125	118.02	6.98	48.69
109	112.65	−3.65	13.30
110	110.69	−0.69	0.48
117	109.23	7.77	60.42
110	107.27	2.73	7.44
98	103.36	−5.36	28.77

(continues)

FROM THE STATISTICIAN *Brendan Heavey*

		SSE	
IQ [Y_i]	**$\hat{Y}$**	**$(Y_i - \hat{Y}_i)$**	**$(Y_i - \hat{Y}_i)^2$**
94	99.94	−5.94	35.32
90	94.08	−4.08	16.64
84	90.17	−6.17	38.08
81	72.58	8.42	70.89

Now, sum the column on the far right to come up with the SSE:

$$SSE = \sum (Y_i - \hat{Y}_i)^2 = 320.03$$

Now we have all the information we need in order to compute R^2. To do so, compute:

$$R^2 = \frac{SSR}{SSTO} = \frac{1599.57}{1919.6} = 0.833$$

The section of a printout from SPSS that pertains to R-squared is shown here:

Model Summary

Model	**R**	**R-Squared**	**Adjusted R-Squared**	**Std. Error of the Estimate**
1	0.913[a]	0.833	0.812	6.32488

[a]Predictors: (Constant), BLL

So, our calculations match . . . hooray!

You will also see the next column, or the **adjusted R-squared**, which is sometimes used to avoid overestimating R^2 (the percentage of variance in the outcome explained by the model), particularly when you have a large number of independent variables with a relatively small sample size. In that case, reporting the adjusted R-squared would be a better idea. The takeaway idea here is this: If you plan to include a larger number of independent variables, you should plan for a larger sample size; otherwise, you are probably overestimating the percentage of variance explained by your regression model (R^2)—and you know the statisticians will not like that!

The **standard error of the estimate** tells you the average amount of error there will be in the predicted outcome (in this case, weight) using this model. (It is the standard deviation of the residuals for those statisticians among you. See the "From the Statistician" titled What

Is a Residual? earlier in this chapter to learn more.) In this example, using both age and height as independent variables, the weight you will predict will be off by an average of approximately 17 pounds. Obviously, you want your prediction to be as accurate as possible, so you would like to see the standard error of the estimate as close to zero as possible.

So now that you know what all of these columns mean, let's go back to the R^2 of 85%, which sounds pretty good. But you know that like all other statistical tests, we still need to look at the p-value to see if it is significant. With multiple regression, you need to see if the R^2 is significant, but you also need to see if each of the independent variables is significant as well. You could have a significant R^2 with an independent variable that really is not adding anything to the regression model, in which case you wouldn't want to keep that variable in your equation.

Okay, so how do we do all of this? Well, let's take it step by step. If I ask SPSS to tell me the **R-squared change**, I can see what happens to the R-squared each time I add another independent variable to the regression model.

Model Summary

Model	R	R-Squared	Adjusted R-Squared	Std. Error of the Estimate	Change Statistics				
					R-Squared Change	F Change	df_1	df_2	Sig. F Change
1	0.656[a]	0.430	0.367	31.24864	0.430	6.788	1	9	0.028
2	0.922[b]	0.850	0.813	16.99823	0.420	22.416	1	8	0.001

[a]Predictors: (Constant), age
[b]Predictors: (Constant), age, height

This output shows me that when I added the variable of age, the R-squared went from 0 to 0.43, and it had a p-value of 0.028, which is significant assuming an alpha of 0.05. When I added height to the model (which now includes age and height as independent variables), the R-squared went from 0.43 to 0.85 (from explaining 43% of the variance to explaining 85% of the variance), or a change of 0.42 (42%), which had a p-value of 0.001, which is also significant at an alpha of 0.05. Adding the second independent variable increased the accuracy of predictions made with this model by increasing the amount of variance accounted for by the model.

If we look at the next table SPSS gives us, you will see an ANOVA table.

ANOVA[a]

Model		Sum of Squares	df	Mean Square	F	Sig.
1	Regression	6628.609	1	6628.609	6.788	0.028[b]
	Residual	8788.300	9	976.478		
	Total	15416.909	10			
2	Regression	13105.391	2	6552.695	22.678	0.001[c]
	Residual	2311.518	8	288.940		
	Total	15416.909	10			

[a]Dependent Variable: Weight
[b]Predictors: (Constant), age
[c]Predictors: (Constant), age, height

In this table you can see the p-value for both the first model (just age included) and the second (age and height included). The first model had a p-value of 0.028, and the second model had a significance level of 0.001.

The last table we see in SPSS shows us the coefficients or the b values in our regression equation.

When we use regression to make predictions, we should look at the column for the unstandardized coefficients (B). First, the B of 584.8 is the constant for our prediction equation. Then you will see the beta coefficients for our independent variables of age and height. This is just the b value in the regression equation. It tells us what a one-unit change in the independent variable will do to the outcome or dependent variable when the other independent variables are held constant. In this example, including both variables in the model gives us $b_1 = 1.712$ and $b_2 = 10.372$. Yikes, we are getting really statistical here—how about a little plain English?

That means, when we control for height, every additional year of age adds 1.71 pounds, and when we control for age, every additional inch of height adds 10.37 pounds. That should make sense—being taller and getting older both tend to add weight. Not a pretty picture but the reality most of us face anyhow. Both age ($p = 0.010$) and height ($p = 0.001$) are significant, which means even when you control for the other, both add to the ability of the model to predict weight. If one of these variables was not significant at this point, it would indicate that when we controlled for the other variables, this variable was not significantly adding to the model or did not increase the ability of the model to make an accurate prediction.

Now it is important to note that the order the researcher chooses to enter the variables and interactions between the variables can affect the significance of the variables in question. There are whole books written on these topics, so I won't discuss them in this chapter. Just suffice it to say, researchers shouldn't just enter a bunch of independent variables into the computer and see which ones look significant without a rationale for why they are doing what they are doing.

	Coefficients[a]						
	Unstandardized Coefficients		Standardized Coefficients			95.0% Confidence Interval for B	
Model	B	Std. Error	Beta	t	Sig.	Lower Bound	Upper Bound
1 (Constant)	93.552	31.582		2.962	0.016	22.108	164.996
age	2.348	0.901	0.656	2.605	0.028	0.309	4.386
2 (Constant)	−584.801	144.305		−4.053	0.004	−917.568	−252.034
age	1.712	0.508	0.478	3.368	0.010	0.540	2.884
height	10.372	2.191	0.672	4.735	0.001	5.320	15.423

[a]Dependent Variable: Weight

In our example, the analysis gives us a regression equation we can then use to predict weight:

$$\text{Weight} = -584 + 1.71(\text{years of age})$$

$$+ 10.37(\text{height in inches}) + \text{error}$$

If a 20-year-old patient was 70 inches tall, you would predict that she might weigh

$$-584 + 17.1(20) + 10.37(70) = 176.1 \text{ pounds}$$

Now I do have to put in one more disclaimer here, which is that making predictions is actually a very complicated process in statistics and what we covered here is really only the first step. For what you need to know at this point, I believe using the word *prediction* is still the best way to explain the topic, but it probably made a few statisticians twitch. Just remember, there is more to come as you go on with your statistics knowledge—such fun to look forward to!

Now there is one last form of regression that I think you should know about: **logistic regression**. Remember that multiple regression involves a continuous dependent variable that is at the interval or ratio level. Logistic regression is used when you have a *categorical* dependent variable with two categories (nominal or ordinal with two categories), such as living or dying. (Multinomial logistic regression can be used when the dependent variable has more than two categories, but it is beyond the scope of this text—whew!) One of the advantages of using logistic regression is that the technique generates an **odds ratio (OR)**, which is the odds or probability of the outcome occurring divided by the odds or probability of the outcome not occurring.

THINKING IT THROUGH

Tests That Control for the Impact of More than One Independent Variable on a Single Dependent Variable

Dependent Variable	Test	Example
Binary (Yes/No)	Logistic regression	Among adolescents who attempt to commit suicide, what is the relationship between alcohol consumption, age, gender, and risk of death? (independent variables: alcohol consumption, age, gender; dependent variable: death [yes/no])*
Continuous variable	Multiple regression	How do parents' education level, income level, and school district rank affect fourth-grade reading scores among impoverished children? (independent variables: parents' education level, income level, and school district rank; dependent variable: reading score at the interval/ratio level)*

*Multiple and logistic regression allow the researcher to examine the effect of multiple independent variables on a single dependent variable. For example, if the researcher believes that maternal age and smoking both have an impact on infant birth weight, the relationship between maternal age and infant birth weight can be seen while controlling for the impact of smoking on infant birth weight.

FROM THE STATISTICIAN *Brendan Heavey*

Methods: Multiple Regression

To tell you the truth, learning how to estimate parameters in a multiple regression model is not worth the time it would take to learn unless you have a little background in linear algebra. If you happen to have a good sense of working with matrices, I would encourage you to take a full course in regression because most of the fundamentals are exceptionally interesting. In this text, however, we're going to assume that the way you will estimate parameters in regression models with multiple independent variables is by setting up the model in a statistical computing package like SPSS and making the computer perform the calculations for you.

Let's say, for instance, we are interested in expanding our study of the effect that blood lead level has on children's IQ. A second variable that we may have some interest in is the IQ of each child's mother. Due to this interest, you might include another question in the study's survey and have data that looks like this:

BLL (mcg/dL)	Mother's IQ	Child's IQ
7	120	125
18	111	109
22	119	110
25	115	117
29	110	110
37	100	98
44	125	94
56	80	90
64	81	84
100	95	81

In this case, we have two independent variables, blood lead level and mother's IQ, and we're interested to see how well we can determine what a child's IQ will be given *both* of these predictors. So, in essence, we want to set up a multiple regression model in SPSS with two independent variables, BLL and mother's IQ, and one dependent variable, child's IQ.

There are two differences in the setup of this model from the one we set up in the last "From the Statistician" feature. First, your data set will have another variable, so it will look like this:

FROM THE STATISTICIAN *Brendan Heavey*

Serum Lead Levels and IQ.

	BII	MothersIQ	IQ
1	7.00	120.00	125.00
2	18.00	111.00	109.00
3	22.00	119.00	110.00
4	25.00	115.00	117.00
5	29.00	110.00	110.00
6	37.00	100.00	98.00
7	44.00	125.00	94.00
8	56.00	80.00	90.00
9	64.00	81.00	84.00
10	100.00	95.00	81.00

Next, when you set up the regression, you will have to add a second variable, MothersIQ, to the list of independent variables, like this:

Adding Independent Variables to a Regression Model using SPSS.

(continues)

FROM THE STATISTICIAN *Brendan Heavey*

The resulting tables will have almost the exact same structure as before but with different data. The only really big difference in the structure of the resulting table is that there will now be three parameters in the Coefficients table, which is reproduced here:

Coefficients[a]

Model	Unstandardized Coefficients		Standardized Coefficients		
	B	Std. Error	Beta	t	Sig.
1 (Constant)	99.624	21.261		4.686	0.002
BLL	−0.420	0.102	−0.784	−4.132	0.004
Mother's IQ	0.180	0.173	0.198	1.042	0.332

[a]Dependent Variable: IQ

Notice there are three parameters: the *y*-intercept or constant, BLL level, and mother's IQ. Each parameter has a coefficient, which is equivalent to what we would call slope if this were a functional relationship. Therefore, this model can be written as:

$$Y = -0.419556X_1 + 0.180322X_2 + 99.624035 + \varepsilon$$

Note: By default, SPSS shows parameter estimates to three decimal places, but for this example, we have performed some magic to get the estimates out to a few more decimals so that the results all tie together.

And you can think of this model as:

$$IQ = -0.419556 \text{ Blood Lead Level} + 0.180322 \ * \text{Mother's IQ} + 99.642035 + \text{Error}$$

So now, if we're interested in what IQ level this model would result in based on a child with a blood lead level of 7 mcg/dL and a mother's IQ of 120, we would plug these two *X*'s into the regression equation and come up with the following result:

$$\hat{Y}\left[IQ\right] = -0.419556 \ * \ 7 + 0.180322 \ * \ 120 + 99.624035$$

$$\hat{Y} = -2.937 + 21.639 + 99.624$$

$$\hat{Y} = 118.33$$

FROM THE STATISTICIAN *Brendan Heavey*

Based on the same logic, we would come up with the following fitted values for our regression function (in the right-most column):

X_1 BLL (mcg/dL)	X_2 Mother's IQ	IQ	$\hat{Y}$
7	120	125	118.33
18	111	109	112.09
22	119	110	111.85
25	115	117	109.87
29	110	110	107.29
37	100	98	102.13
44	125	94	103.70
56	80	90	90.55
64	81	84	87.38
100	95	81	74.80

Now, something really interesting: Once you calculate all of the $\hat{Y}$'s, the rest of the model equations are exactly the same as in the single predictor case:

$$SSTO = \sum (Y_i - \overline{Y})^2$$

Here are all the numbers we'll need to calculate SSTO:

Y_i	$\overline{Y}$	$(Y_i - \overline{Y})^2$	$(Y_i - \overline{Y})^2$
125	101.8	23.2	538.24
109	101.8	7.2	51.84
110	101.8	8.2	67.24
117	101.8	15.2	231.04
110	101.8	8.2	67.24
98	101.8	−3.8	14.44
94	101.8	−7.8	60.84
90	101.8	−11.8	139.24
84	101.8	−17.8	316.84
81	101.8	−20.8	432.64

(continues)

FROM THE STATISTICIAN *Brendan Heavey*

Now, sum the right-most column:

$$SSTO = 1919.6$$

Next, SSR's formula:

$$SSR = \sum (\hat{Y}_i - \overline{Y})^2$$

And all the data we'll need:

$\hat{Y}_i$	$\overline{Y}$	$(\hat{Y}_i - \overline{Y})$	$(\hat{Y}_i - \overline{Y})^2$
118.33	101.8	16.53	273.11
112.09	101.8	10.29	105.84
111.85	101.8	10.05	101.05
109.87	101.8	8.07	65.16
107.29	101.8	5.49	30.17
102.13	101.8	0.33	0.11
103.70	101.8	1.90	3.63
90.55	101.8	−11.25	126.46
87.38	101.8	−14.42	207.98
74.80	101.8	−27.00	729.05

Sum the right-most column:

$$SSR = 1642.535$$

SSE's formula is:

$$SSE = \sum (Y_i - \hat{Y}_i)$$

All the data:

Y_i	$\hat{Y}_i$	$(\hat{Y}_i - \overline{Y})$	$(Y_i - \hat{Y}_i)^2$
125	118.33	6.67	44.54
109	112.09	−3.09	9.54
110	111.85	−1.85	3.43
117	109.87	7.13	50.80
110	107.29	2.71	7.33
98	102.13	−4.13	17.08
94	103.70	−9.70	94.17
90	90.55	−0.55	0.31
84	87.38	−3.38	11.42
81	74.80	6.20	38.45

Sum the right-most column:

$$SSE = 277.065$$

Which is great because that's what the output from SPSS tells us in the ANOVA table for this model:

ANOVA[a]

Model	Sum of Squares	df	Mean Square	F	Sig.
1 Regression	1642.535	2	821.268	20.749	0.001[b]
Residual	277.065	7	39.581		
Total	1919.600	9			

[a]Dependent Variable: IQ
[b]Predictors: (Constant), MothersIQ, BLL

(continues)

FROM THE STATISTICIAN *Brendan Heavey*

Now, let's examine the resulting R^2. We could calculate it ourselves using the same equation as before, substituting the values in the ANOVA table for SSTO and SSR:

$$R^2 = \frac{SSR}{SSTO}$$

$$= \frac{1642.535}{1919.600}$$

$$= 0.856$$

Or we could just look at the first table produced by SPSS for this model:

Model Summary

Model	R	R-Squared	Adjusted R-Squared	Std. Error of the Estimate
1	0.925[a]	0.856	0.814	6.29132

[a]Predictors: (Constant), MothersIQ, BLL

Finally, let's look back at the R^2 value from the model with one predictor variable:

Model Summary

Model	R	R-Squared	Adjusted R-Squared	Std. Error of the Estimate
1	0.913[a]	0.833	0.812	6.32488

[a]Predictors: (Constant), BLL

Notice that our R^2 went from 0.833 to 0.856 just by adding a second predictor. An R^2 that results from a model with multiple independent variables will always be greater than or equal to the R^2 from any of the models resulting from fewer of these same independent variables. Said a different way, when adding more and more predictors, R^2 will never go down.

SUMMARY

Regression analysis is a statistical procedure that allows us to develop a regression equation that we can use to infer or predict future events. There are several types of regression. In this chapter we discussed linear regression, multiple regression, and logistic regression. Linear regression analyzes the relationship between a single independent variable and a single interval- or ratio-level dependent variable. The slope (*b*) of the linear regression equation tells us how much the predicted value of the dependent variable changes when there is a one-unit change in the independent variable. The residual is the prediction error or how far away from the prediction line the actual data points fall.

When researchers want to predict how two or more variables affect a dependent variable, they may use multiple regression, where the values of the regression coefficients (*b*) show the change in the dependent variable for a one-unit increase in the independent variable with which it is associated. Each regression model has a corresponding *R*-squared, which tells you how much of the variance in the

dependent variable (outcome) is explained by the independent variables you have included in the model or equation. When sample size is small, researchers sometimes report the adjusted *R*-squared to avoid overestimating the amount of variance in the dependent variable explained by the independent variables in the equation. The *R*-squared change tells you the additional variance in the dependent variable accounted for when you add another independent variable. Make sure the *R*-squared change is statistically significant if you want to increase the accuracy of your prediction equation.

There will always be some error involved in any prediction (yes—even yours!), and with multiple regression we see this estimated by the standard error of the estimate. Researchers try to make the standard error of the estimate as small as possible, obviously trying to make their predictions as accurate as possible.

The last form of regression we discussed was logistic regression, which is used when the outcome or dependent variable is binary, such as for mortality. Logistic regression lets researchers report an odds ratio that tells them the odds or probability of the outcome event occurring in one group versus another.

CHAPTER 12 REVIEW QUESTIONS

Questions 1–4: Mosfeldt et al. (2012) collected data on 792 patients age 60 or over who were admitted to a hospital in Denmark with a hip fracture between 2008 and 2010. They reported that an elevated creatinine level upon hospital admission for a hip fracture (>90 mmol/L for women and >105 mmol/L for men) is associated with an almost threefold increase in mortality risk.

1. What is the independent variable? What level of measurement is it?

2. What is the dependent variable? What level of measurement is it?

3. What type of sample is this? Is it a probability or nonprobability sample?

4. These researchers chose to use a regression model. Should they perform a linear regression, multiple regression, or logistic regression? Why?

Questions 5–10: In another study, researchers randomly selected five hospitals with orthopedic units in the United States and collected data from all the male patients over age 60 admitted for hip fracture. The researchers then report that admission levels of creatinine and hemoglobin can be used to predict the number of days the patient will need to stay in the hospital.

5. What would be the independent variables? What level are they?

6. What would be the dependent variable? What level is it?

7. What type of sampling method is this? Is it probability or nonprobability sampling?

8. Why might these researchers have chosen to exclude those admitted with a hip fracture who are younger than 60?

9. Would it be appropriate to use these results to predict the length of stay for female patients over age 60 admitted with hip fractures? Why or why not?

10. If these researchers had already established that a causative relationship existed between these variables and asked you for a statistics consultation, what would you tell them is the appropriate regression technique to apply? Explain your answer.

Questions 11–18: Assume that age and academic knowledge (graded exam: 0–100%) have been shown to be related to health knowledge (knowledge questionnaire score: 0–100%) among teens. A nurse researcher would like to use the data she has collected from a random sample of 118 teens living in urban centers of New York to predict their health knowledge. She enters the data she has from their academic knowledge test and their ages into SPSS and formulates the following tables from the multiple regression option:

Variables Entered/Removed.[a]

Model[b]	Variables Entered	Variables Removed	Method
1	academic_knowledge, age		Enter

[a]Dependent Variable: health_knowledge
[b]All requested variables entered.

Model Summary

					Change Statistics				
Model	R	R-Squared	Adjusted R-Squared	Std. Error of the Estimate	R-Squared Change	F Square Change	df₁	df₂	Sig. F Change
1	0.864[a]	0.747	0.743	2.13687	0.747	167.056	2	113	0.000

[a]Predictors: (Constant), academic_knowledge, age

ANOVA[a]

Model	Sum of Squares	df	Mean Square	F	Sig.
1 Regression	1525.629	2	762.814	167.056	0.000[b]
Residual	515.983	113	4.566		
Total	2041.612	115			

[a]Dependent Variable: health_knowledge
[b]Predictors: (Constant), academic_knowledge, age

Coefficients[a]

	Unstandardized Coefficients		Standardized Coefficients		
Model	B	Std. Error	Beta	t	Sig.
1 (Constant)	41.891	3.294		12.716	0.000
age	2.711	0.157	0.853	17.322	0.000
academic_knowledge	−0.023	0.029	0.039	0.791	0.430

[a]Dependent Variable: health_knowledge

11. According to the SPSS output, what percentage of the variance in health knowledge is explained by age and academic knowledge?

12. Is the *R*-squared significant? Explain your answer.

13. Should the nurse researcher include both independent variables in her final model? Explain your answer.

14. If the nurse researcher includes both independent variables in her prediction equation, her predicted health knowledge score will be incorrect by an average of how many points?

15. According to this model, every 1-year increase in age results in what change in the health knowledge score?

16. Using this model, if a 15-year-old scored 70 on his academic knowledge exam, what would you expect him to score on his health knowledge exam?

17. What type of sample is this?

18. A researcher working with military officers would like to use the data he has collected from them to predict their health knowledge score based on this research. Would this be an appropriate application of this prediction equation? Why or why not?

Questions 19–21: The nurse researcher in questions 11–18 examined her SPSS output and decided to drop the second independent variable (score on the academic knowledge exam) from her model. Doing so resulted in the following SPSS output:

Variables Entered/Removed[a]

Model	Variables Entered	Variables Removed	Method
1	age[b]	.	Enter

[a]Dependent Variable: health_knowledge
[b]All requested variables entered.

Model Summary

Model	R	R-Squared	Adjusted R-Squared	Std. Error of the Estimate
1	0.864[a]	0.746	0.744	2.13337

[a]Predictors: (Constant), age

ANOVA[a]

Model	Sum of Squares	df	Mean Square	F	Sig.
1 Regression	1522.769	1	1522.769	334.582	0.000[b]
Residual	518.844	114	4.551		
Total	2041.612	115			

[a]Dependent Variable: health_knowledge
[b]Predictors: (Constant), age

Coefficients[a]

Model	Unstandardized Coefficients		Standardized Coefficients	t	Sig.
	B	Std. Error	Beta		
1 (Constant)	39.890	2.108		18.920	0.000
age	2.746	0.150	0.864	18.292	0.000

[a]Dependent Variable: health_knowledge

19. Does this model explain more or less of the variance in the health knowledge score? Is this a large change? Does that make sense?

20. In which model is the predicted outcome more accurate?

21. Using this prediction equation, if a 15-year-old scored 70 on his academic knowledge exam, what would you predict he would score on his health knowledge exam?

Questions 22–25: This sample includes 9 teens age 14, 12 teens age 15, 25 teens age 16, 27 teens age 17, and 45 teens age 18.

22. Show this frequency distribution graphically.

23. What level of measurement is age in this example?

24. Calculate all appropriate measures of central tendency for this variable.

25. Is age normally distributed in this sample? Explain your answer.

Questions 26–28: Khan, Sobki, and Alhomida (2015) examined 75 patients to assess the association between fasting blood sugar (FBS) measured in mmol/l and glycosylated hemoglobin (HbA1c) levels measured as a percentage and reported the following regression equation, which can be used to estimate an HbA1C level from a FBS level.

$$HbA1c = 0.387 \,(FBS) + 4.855$$

26. From this equation you know that an increase of 1 unit in FBS is associated with what change in HbA1c?

27. The researchers also examined the independent variable of gender but did not include this variable in the final regression equation. Why do you think gender was not included in the final regression model?

_____

_____

28. The researchers report that ethnicity was not measured in this study but has been reported to be significant in other similar studies. If the study were repeated and ethnicity was included, and if none of the independent variables was then significant, we would know the original study that reported FBS was significantly related to HbA1c had made what type of error?

_____

_____

Questions 29 and 30: The Khan et al. (2015) study also reported the following regression equation and reported that HbA1c could also be used to predict FBS.

$$FBS = 1.33(HbA1c) - 2.528$$

29. If HbA1c is 8%, what would be the predicted in mmol/l of FBS?

_____

_____

30. If HbA1c increases by 2%, what would be the predicted change in FBS?

_____

_____

Research Application Article

Here's an example of how multiple regression can be useful in a research study. Sometimes it helps you understand the concept when you see it applied in a real-life scenario. In a study completed by Tussey et al. (2015), laboring women who had received an epidural were randomized into two groups and compared. One group was given routine care; the experimental group was provided with a peanut-shaped exercise ball. The ball was used to support maternal positioning that promoted spinal flexion; fetal head rotation; and widening of the pelvic inlet, outlet, and intertuberous diameter. Answer the following questions regarding this study.

Tussey, C. M., Botsios, E., Gerkin, R. D., Kelly, L. A., Gamez, J., & Mensik, J. (2015). Reducing length of labor and cesarean surgery rate using a peanut ball for women laboring with an epidural. *The Journal of Perinatal Education, 24*(1), 16–24. doi:10.1891/1058-1243.24.1.16

1. What was the purpose of the study?
2. What are the outcome variables in this study?
3. What level of measurement are the outcome variables?
4. Look at Table 1 in the article. Despite randomization, there were significant differences in demographic characteristics noted between the control and experimental groups. Which characteristics had significant differences between the two groups?
5. Look at Table 2 in the article. Was there a significant difference in the average length of the second stage of labor between the two groups? How do you know?
6. Look at Table 2 in the article. Was there a significant difference in the number of cesarean sections between the two groups? How do you know?

7. When looking at the differences in these outcome variables, length of the second stage of labor and mode of delivery, two different tests were used. Why?

8. When offering the option of using a peanut-shaped exercise ball to your patient, her mother expresses concern that this type of positioning might increase the risk of the baby being born with a nuchal cord. Use the results of Table 2 in the article to address this concern.

9. The researchers report that parity (number of births) and cervical dilation were different between the two groups. Because these factors can have an impact on the outcome variables and were not controlled for in the sample selection, what technique might you consider that would allow you to include the impact they may have on the outcome?

10. Look at Table 3 in the article. The researchers decided to perform univariate analyses of each independent variable and each of the three outcome variables. Which independent variables were significantly associated with the risk of a cesarean delivery?

11. Look at Table 4 in the article. The researchers included the independent variables that were significantly associated with the outcomes variables in the univariate analysis in their multiple regression analysis. They kept those with a $p < 0.05$ in their final multivariate regression models. Controlling for the other independent variables, which independent variables were significantly associated with the length of the first stage of labor in the multivariate regression model?

12. Look at Table 4 in the article. Explain the beta coefficient for cervical dilation.

13. Look at Table 4 in the article. The researchers included the independent variables that were significantly associated with the outcomes variables in the univariate analysis in their multiple regression analysis. They kept those with a $p < 0.05$ in their final multivariate regression models. Controlling for the other independent variables, which independent variables were significantly associated with the length of the second stage of labor in the multivariate regression model?

14. If the finding about the relationship between using the peanut-shaped ball and the length of the first stage of labor was incorrect, what type of error would it be? What would be the most likely cause of this type of error?

15. The researchers discuss in their Power Analysis section that they estimated the effect size from the results of a small pilot study. If the impact of the use of a ball on the length of the first stage of labor was actually overestimated in the pilot study, how would this affect the estimate of the effect size used by the researchers? How would the effect size they used affect the sample size selected? How might this affect the results?

16. The researchers use a logistic regression model rather than a multivariate regression model to assess the delivery mode outcome. Why is this?

17. Is the use of the ball significantly associated with the risk of a cesarean delivery? How do you know?

18. Is the use of the ball a protective effect or risk factor for a cesarean section delivery?

19. Using the ball was significantly associated with a decrease in the length of the second stage of labor. Although this outcome is usually a positive result, nurses should avoid using this intervention for what group of patients?

20. Based on the results in this study, what happened with this nurse-led intervention?

ANSWERS TO ODD-NUMBERED CHAPTER 12 REVIEW QUESTIONS

1. Creatinine level, interval/ratio

3. Convenience, nonprobability

5. Creatinine levels upon admission and hemoglobin levels upon admission, interval/ratio level

7. Cluster sampling, probability sampling

9. No, the sample includes only men, so it is not representative of a population of women.

11. R-squared $= 74.7\%$, adjusted R-squared $= 74.3\%$

13. No, beta for age is 2.711 with a significant p-value ($p = 0.000$), whereas the b for academic knowledge is -0.023, which is insignificant ($p = 0.43$).

15. An increase of 2.711 points (unstandardized age coefficient $= 2.711$)

17. Random or probability sample

19. The model explains slightly less of the variance in the health knowledge score. (R-squared changes from 0.747 to 0.746.) This is not a large change, which makes sense because an independent variable was eliminated in this model, but it was an insignificant independent variable, so the change should be small.

21. $81.08 = 39.89 + 2.746(15)$

23. Interval

25. No, the mean, median, and mode are not equal; therefore, we know the sample is not normally distributed.

27. Gender was not a significant independent variable and was not included to minimize the prediction error

29. $1.33(8) - 2.528 = 8.112$

Answers to Research Application Article

1. To determine if the use of the peanut-shaped exercise ball affected the length and method of delivery.

3. Length of labor is interval, and mode of birth is nominal.

5. Yes, the average length of the second stage of labor was 21.3 in the peanut ball group (PBG) and 43.5 in the Control (C) group. A t-test was completed with a p-value of 0.006, which is less than alpha, so the difference is statistically significant.

7. The length of the second stage of labor was an interval-level variable, so the researchers could determine a mean value and look for differences in the mean value using a t-test. The outcome variable of mode of delivery was only at the nominal level (vaginal/cesarean); thus, no mean is available, and the appropriate test to compare the two groups is a chi-square.

9. A multivariate regression would allow you to see how individual independent variables affect the outcome variable while controlling for the impact of other independent variables.

11. Maternal age ($p = 0.011$), cervical dilation ($p < 0.001$), nulliparous status ($p < 0.001$)

13. It was close to being significant ($p = 0.053$), but it was not less than alpha, so it was not significant.

15. Type two—missing a relationship that really exists, which is usually caused by an underpowered study that did not have a large enough sample to detect a significant difference that really exists

17. The outcome variable (delivery mode) is at the nominal level (vaginal/cesarean). A logistic regression is the appropriate test to assess the relationship between multiple independent variables and a single binary outcome variable.

19. It is a protective factor that significantly decreases the risk of a cesarean section.

21. It was implemented for all appropriate patients in the study hospital and then in all of the labor units in the hospital system. Great job nurse researchers!

RELATIVE RISK, ODDS RATIO, AND ATTRIBUTABLE RISK

MAKING THE PUBLIC ANNOUNCEMENT

OBJECTIVES

By the end of this chapter students will be able to:

- Define epidemiology.

- Compare and contrast the three major study designs used in epidemiology, and evaluate the strengths and weaknesses of each.

- Compare and contrast incidence data and prevalence data.

- Explain why relative risk is a helpful measure.

- Write null and alternative hypotheses that demonstrate an understanding of relative risk (RR) and the odds ratio (OR).

- Formulate a 2 × 2 table from a given data set.

- Calculate incidence rates, relative risk, and odds ratios.

- Interpret relative risks and odds ratios of less than one, equal to one, and greater than one.

- Evaluate whether it is appropriate to calculate a relative risk or an odds ratio from three nursing research proposals.

- Calculate the attributable risk for the exposed group, and interpret it for the exposed group in statistical terms and in plain English.

- Calculate attack rates, and determine the likely source of an outbreak.

- Prepare a public health headline that states attributable risk results in language the general population will understand.

- Critique a current nursing research article that utilizes odds ratios, and interpret the results statistically and in plain English.
- Prepare a public health report using odds ratio results in language the general public will understand.

- Interpret Statistical Package for the Social Sciences (SPSS) output, and determine whether a given relative risk and odds ratio are significant. Explain these results statistically and in plain English.

KEY TERMS

Attack rate

The incidence rate in the exposed group or the number of cases divided by all those exposed to a particular agent.

Attributable risk for the exposed group (AR$_e$)

The amount of a disease or an outcome in an exposed group that is due to a particular exposure.

Case control study

A study design that starts with the outcome of interest and looks back to determine exposure.

Cohort study

A prospective design that follows a group of individuals over time to see who develops the outcome of interest.

Cross-sectional study

A study design that collects the data about exposure and outcome at the same time.

Epidemiology

The study of the distribution of disease.

Incidence cases

The number of new cases that occur among a sample during the duration of the study.

Odds ratio (OR)

An approximation of the relative risk using prevalence data (the odds that a case was exposed divided by the odds that a control was exposed).

Prevalence cases

Those cases that already exist in a population.

Protective effect

When an exposure helps prevent a disease (a significant relative risk of less than one).

Relative risk (RR)

The incidence rate in the exposed sample divided by the incidence rate of those not exposed.

Relative risk of one

No association between the exposure and the illness.

Risk factor

An exposure associated with increased rates of disease.

Risk ratio

Another name for relative risk.

EPIDEMIOLOGY

Nursing is overlapping more and more with **epidemiology**, which is actually the study of the distribution of disease (Gordis, 2000). (Many people, including many who should know better, have no idea what epidemiology is. Although I have a doctorate in epidemiology, on multiple occasions I have been introduced as an endocrinologist!) Epidemiologists like to see how disease is distributed and then ask the age-old question: Why? Some of the tools we use to examine this question in the public health arena are becoming more and more popular in nursing research, so I am going to make sure you are ready to combine what you know as a nurse with what you can learn about epidemiology in this chapter.

STUDY DESIGNS USED IN EPIDEMIOLOGY

There are basically three types of epidemiological studies (and many hybrid versions of them that you don't have to worry about right now):

- Cohort study
- Case control study
- Cross-sectional study

COHORT STUDY

A **cohort study** is a prospective design that follows a group of individuals over time to see who develops the outcome of interest. For example, you might follow the nurses at your hospital to see which, if any, develop osteoporosis. In a cohort study, you start by measuring exposure, and then you monitor for outcomes. In this example study, the exposure you are measuring is consumption of dairy products, and you are monitoring for the outcome of osteoporosis.

You also have to eliminate the **prevalence cases**, that is, the nurses who already have the disease you wish to study. Then you conduct an initial survey of the remaining nurses to see what they eat and drink, whether they smoke, whether they lift patients regularly, what unit they work on, how many hours they sleep, and so on. You then monitor the group for 40 years and see who develops osteoporosis, your outcome of interest. You can also look at multiple exposures (diet, smoking, lifting, sleeping, etc.) and determine which, if any, are associated with developing osteoporosis later in life.

One of the advantages of this type of study is that you can monitor for **incidence cases**, which are the new cases that occur among your sample during the duration of your study. That enables you to calculate something called a **relative risk (RR)**, which is the incidence rate in the exposed sample divided by the incidence rate of those not exposed. The relative risk is also sometimes referred to as the **risk ratio**. Let's try calculating a relative risk. The tricky part is setting up your 2×2 table correctly with the given information. I always suggest having several blank 2×2 tables (**Figure 13-1**) ready when you have homework or tests coming up, to make sure you have everything ready when you need it.

Let's work this example through together. Suppose there are 1,000 people in a town that was recently devastated by a hurricane. Half the town (500 people) became sick within 2 weeks of the hurricane. It turns out that, of the half who got sick, 468 were living in an area where the local water supply was compromised and high bacteria levels were detected. Sixty-three of those who did not get sick lived in this same area with contaminated water. If we want to calculate the RR of becoming sick when "exposed" to living in the area with contaminated water, we will start by filling in the appropriate cells in our 2×2 table.

FIGURE 13-1

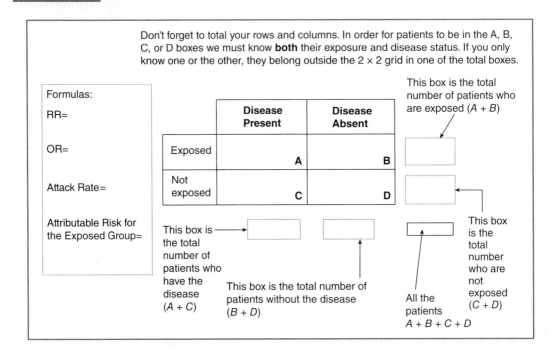

Start with the first bit of data you have—the total number of people:

	Disease Present	Disease Absent	Total
Exposed	A	B	
Not exposed	C	D	
			1,000

A = subjects with the exposure and the disease

B = subjects with the exposure and without the disease

C = subjects without the exposure but with the disease

D = subjects without the exposure and without the disease

Then the question tells you that half of the town gets sick, so fill that in:

	Disease Present	Disease Absent	Total
Exposed			
Not exposed			
	500		1,000

This means half of the town does not get sick:

	Disease Present	Disease Absent	Total
Exposed			
Not exposed			
	500	500	1,000

You are then told that, of the half that got sick, 468 lived in the exposure area, so fill that in:

	Disease Present	Disease Absent	Total
Exposed	468		
Not exposed	32		
	500	500	1,000

In other words, of those who got sick, 32 were not living in the exposure region because the column must add up to the total number who got sick, or 500.

You are then told that 63 of those who did not get sick lived in the exposure area, so fill in that cell:

	Disease Present	Disease Absent	Total
Exposed	468	63	
Not exposed	32		
	500	500	1,000

Now all that is left to complete your table is a bit of math. The Disease Absent column has to add up to the total at the bottom of 500 (total number who are not sick), so you know there were 437 people who were not living in the exposure area and did not get sick.

	Disease Present	Disease Absent	Total
Exposed	468	63	
Not exposed	32	437	
	500	500	1,000

Then, add up the rows to get your totals in the last columns for those exposed (468 + 63) and those not exposed (32 + 437):

	Disease Present	Disease Absent	Total
Exposed	468	63	531
Not exposed	32	437	469
	500	500	1,000

The last step is to calculate the relative risk, which is the incidence rate in the exposed group divided by the incidence rate in the unexposed group:

$$RR = \frac{\dfrac{A}{A+B}}{\dfrac{C}{C+D}}$$

A = subjects with the exposure and the disease
B = subjects with the exposure and without the disease
C = subjects without the exposure but with the disease
D = subjects without the exposure and without the disease

$$RR = \frac{468 \,/\, 531}{32 \,/\, 469} = \frac{0.88}{0.07} = 12.57$$

In plain English, this means that the group that lived in the area with the contaminated water was 12.57 times as likely to become sick compared to those who lived elsewhere in the town. If the relative risk is greater than one, the group that was exposed has a higher incidence rate than the group that was not. Thus, exposure to the area with the contaminated water may be a risk factor for developing the disease (we still don't know if it is a statistically significant risk factor until we see the *p*-value or the confidence interval, which we will discuss later in the chapter).

Let's look at one more example. In a sample of 300 nurses, you found that, of the 100 nurses who consumed three servings of dairy products daily, only 4 developed osteoporosis. At the same time, among the 200 nurses who did not consume three servings of dairy products daily, 20 developed osteoporosis. We can make a 2 × 2 table to help sort out the results (see **Table 13-1**).

The incidence cases are all the nurses who developed osteoporosis during the 40-year span of your study: $A + C = 24$. The incidence rate is simply the incidence cases divided by the whole sample times 100: in this case, $24 \div 300 \times 100 = 8\%$. This calculation tells you that 8% of your sample developed osteoporosis during the course of your study. You now need to compare the incidence in the exposed sample to the incidence in the nonexposed sample or the relative risk (RR). The formula is:

$$RR = \frac{\dfrac{A}{A+B}}{\dfrac{C}{C+D}}$$

where

A = subjects with the exposure and the disease
B = subjects with the exposure and without the disease
C = subjects without the exposure but with the disease
D = subjects without the exposure and without the disease

The calculation in this case is:

$$RR = \frac{4 \,/\, 100}{20 \,/\, 200} = \frac{0.04}{0.1} \text{ , or } 40\%$$

The interpretation of this result is that those who were exposed (consumed three servings of dairy a day) were less than half as likely (40% as likely) to develop osteoporosis later in life as those who were not exposed (didn't consume three servings of dairy daily). In this case, the exposure may have had a **protective effect** on disease development.

Interpretations of relative risk include the following:

- A relative risk of less than one means the group that was exposed had fewer cases

TABLE 13-1	**Consumption of Three Dairy Products (Exposure) and Osteoporosis Disease (Disease)**		
	Disease	**No Disease**	**Total**
Exposed	$A = 4$	$B = 96$	$A + B = 100$
Not exposed*	$C = 20$	$D = 180$	$C + D = 200$
Total	$A + C = 24$	$B + D = 276$	$A + B + C + D = 300$

*Did not consume three dairy products a day.

develop (lower incidence) than the group that was not exposed. This means the exposure may be a protective factor, much like a vaccine, that helps prevent disease development.

- A **relative risk of one** indicates that there is no association between the exposure and the illness. For example, you may have found that consuming two cups of fruit juice had no effect on future osteoporosis development; this finding would be reflected by a relative risk of approximately one. The incidence of the disease is the same in the group that was exposed and in the group that was not. There is no relationship between the exposure and the disease.

- If the relative risk is greater than one, the group that was exposed has a higher incidence rate than the group that was not. Thus, the exposure may be a **risk factor** for the development of the disease. For example, let's say that you found in your study that the relative risk for smokers was 5.0. This number means that the incidence rate for osteoporosis was five times higher for smokers than for nonsmokers. Put a little differently, those who smoked were five times as likely to develop osteoporosis.

Don't forget that even with a relative risk as high as 5.0, you still need to see whether the number is statistically significant. Statistical significance of the relative risk is once again determined by the *p*-value of the associated chi-square test. You always need to check the *p*-value. However, sometimes you will see a relative risk reported without the *p*-value stated explicitly. Instead you will see something called confidence intervals (CIs) or confidence limits (CLs) (see **Figure 13-2**). When you are given the RR that is determined in the study

(using a sample) without a *p*-value and a 95% confidence limit is reported, it just means that the researcher is 95% sure that the actual RR *in the population* is between these two numbers. (The 95% confidence limits are typically applied and reflect an alpha of 0.05. If there is an alpha of 0.10, you may see 90% confidence limits or intervals reported.) How you interpret the significance of the *p*-value in this situation is not terribly complicated, so let's try it. If there is an RR of 2.3 with a 95% confidence interval of 1.2–3.5 in your study, interpreting this value would just mean you are 95% sure that the RR in the population (remember your sample just estimates it) is between 1.2 and 3.5. Anywhere in this range, you see a higher rate of disease in the exposed group. Even at the low end, the exposed group is 1.2 times as likely to develop the disease when compared to the unexposed group. This is a situation where the *p*-value is less than alpha, and there is a significant relationship between the exposure and the disease; the exposure is a risk factor for the development of the disease anywhere on the continuum of the confidence limits. Thus, there is a significant difference in the incidence rates between the two groups and thus a statistically significant RR.

However, if the confidence interval or limits are 0.23–3.59, you can see that the confidence interval's lower value is below 1 and the upper value is greater than 1. Think about what this means, and it will make sense. In this case, you are 95% certain that the actual RR in the population is between 0.23 and 3.59. If the actual RR is at the bottom end of the confidence interval, it would be around 0.23, and the exposed group would have less of the disease than the nonexposed group (protective exposure). If the RR in the population is 1 (which is included in the 95% confidence interval), then there is no relationship between the exposure and the disease because

FIGURE 13-2   **Relative Risk.**

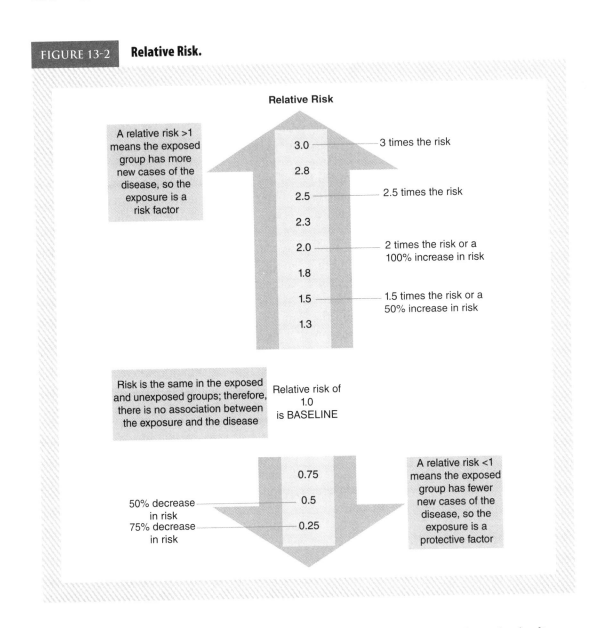

the disease levels are the same in both the exposed and nonexposed groups. If the RR in the population is near the top of the 95% CI, then it would be around 3.5, which would mean the exposed group had higher levels of the disease (the exposure is a risk factor). So you are 95% certain that the exposure is either a protective factor, not related, or a risk factor for the disease. How wishy-washy is that? That is how you know you do not have a significant p-value. Whenever the confidence limits include the value of 1, you have an insignificant p-value because you are not certain enough to know whether there is a relationship or not. Remember, an RR of one means no relationship, which is your null hypothesis. If the confidence limits include the possibility of the null hypothesis, you cannot reject the null hypothesis, which means the *p*-value is greater than your identified alpha and you do not have a statistically significant result. If you want to think about this further, take a moment to review the following section: FTS: Confidence Limits.

FROM THE STATISTICIAN *Brendan Heavey*

Confidence Intervals
Confidence Limits

I love to eat! It's one of my favorite things to do on earth. I also love to grill, which is convenient given my love of eating. One of my favorite things to eat is hot dogs—they are tasty and difficult to grill improperly. My 7-year-old nephew also loves to eat hot dogs. In fact, we share such a love of hot dogs that I decided to study our eating habits this year.

I started by collecting data on our combined number of hot dogs consumed per sitting for a year. I thought I'd show my nephew a little about what statistical inference means, so I showed him only five randomly selected sets of data and asked him to guess what the average total of hot dogs consumed per sitting would be for the whole year. Here's the data:

Sitting	Me	My Nephew	Combined Hot Dogs Consumed
1	3 hot dogs	5 hot dogs	8
2	5 hot dogs	6 hot dogs	11
3	3 hot dogs	3 hot dogs	6
4	2 hot dogs	4 hot dogs	6
5	3 hot dogs	5 hot dogs	8

What kind of estimate can we come up with for average hot dogs consumed per sitting for the whole year using this data?

Here's how a statistician would approach this problem. We know the mean for this sample was:

$$\frac{8 + 11 + 6 + 6 + 8}{5} = \frac{39}{5} = 7.8$$

This is a single number, sometimes called a point estimate, that is a reasonably good guess for the whole year if this sample is the only data we have to base our estimate on. However, this is one sample that doesn't necessarily represent the actual population mean perfectly. Given what we know about the central limit theorem and the normal distribution, is there a more precise estimate we can come up with?

(continues)

FROM THE STATISTICIAN *Brendan Heavey*

If we are okay with a few assumptions about our data, we can figure out an interval or range that the mean most likely fell into at the end of the year. This range is called a confidence interval.

A confidence interval is reported as two numbers that represent the high and low values of a range around our point estimate. We could calculate many different kinds of confidence intervals. In this text, we will deal strictly with 95% confidence intervals from small samples.

In this example, the lower *confidence limit* turns out to be:

$$CL_l = 7.8 - 5.2 = 2.6$$

While our upper *confidence limit* turns out to be:

$$CL_U = 7.8 + 5.2 = 13$$

What does a confidence interval tell us? Here is a (potentially) oversimplified answer: We are 95% confident that our population parameter (i.e., average hot dogs per sitting for the whole year) falls between these two numbers.

In my experience, the majority of clinicians understand confidence intervals using this interpretation, which is fine in a clinical setting. This interpretation is a little oversimplified, however, and if you're going to venture into a career in research, you should try to understand the concept in a more nuanced manner.

Here is the more appropriate way to think of confidence intervals: If we were to sample randomly from a population many times and calculate a 95% CI on each of those samples, the true population parameter would fall inside our calculated range 95% of the time. In this case, if we took 1,000 random samples of hot dogs eaten per sitting and calculated 95% confidence intervals on each of those samples, the true annual mean would fall inside about 950 of the intervals we calculated.

Let's look at the formula for a confidence interval:

$$\text{Sample Mean} \pm \text{Critical Value} * \frac{\text{Sample Std. Dev}}{\sqrt{\text{Sample Size}}}$$

This looks little daunting, but there are really only two parts of this formula I want you to concentrate on. First, sample size is in the denominator, or the third term, which means that sample size is inversely proportional to confidence interval size. In other words, if we kept all variables the same but added more samples to our estimate, the confidence interval size would decrease. This is probably the trickiest thing you'll have to learn about a confidence interval. Try to remember it this way: The larger the confidence interval size, the less confidence you have in a point estimate.

The second thing to know about confidence intervals is that they are the complement of alpha level. Thus, if you add confidence interval size and alpha level together, you get 1, or 100%. If you build a confidence interval with an alpha level of .05, you are building a 95% confidence interval. If you change your alpha level to .1, you will have a 90% confidence interval.

FROM THE STATISTICIAN *Brendan Heavey*

Methods: Confidence Intervals

Methods

Let's discuss the details of how to calculate a 95% confidence interval around a mean. Let's say that you are involved in an early-stage cancer clinical trial that has performed blood tests on five patients. Their serum creatinine clearance levels are listed in the table below.

Serum Creatinine Clearance
115 mL/min
105 mL/min
96 mL/min
117 mL/min
111 mL/min

We are interested in calculating a 95% confidence interval of the serum creatinine clearance level of patients in the population of interest. Here is the formula for a 95% confidence interval:

$$\overline{x} \pm t_{n-1}^{*} * \frac{s}{\sqrt{n}}$$

where:

$\overline{x}$ is the sample mean

t_{n-1}^{*} is the critical value

s is the sample standard deviation

n is the sample size

So, in this case,

$$\overline{x} = \frac{115 + 105 + 96 + 117 + 111}{5} = 108.8$$

$$\sqrt{n} = \sqrt{5} = 2.24$$

$$s = \sqrt{\frac{\Sigma\left(x - \overline{x}\right)^2}{n-1}}$$

$$= \sqrt{\frac{\left(115 - 108.8\right)^2 + \left(105 - 108.8\right)^2 + \left(96 - 108.8\right)^2 + \left(117 - 108.8\right)^2 + \left(111 - 108.8\right)^2}{5 - 1}} = 8.5$$

(continues)

FROM THE STATISTICIAN *Brendan Heavey*

The critical value, t_{n-1}^*, turns out to be a more difficult task. For many years, statisticians relied on statistical charts to figure out what value to use; however, you can now use an Excel function to get the value. The function to use is TINV. This function has two arguments, the first is the alpha level of the test, and the second is the degrees of freedom. Degrees of freedom are simply $N-1$.

In our case, we enter the following into a cell in Excel:

$$= \text{TINV} (.05, 4)$$

which results in:

$$2.776$$

Therefore, our 95% confidence interval can be calculated as:

$$108.8 \pm 2.776 * \frac{8.5}{2.24} = 108.8 \pm 10.54$$

$$= \{98.26, 119.34\}$$

This is the 95% confidence interval for this sample. If we took 999 more random samples of serum creatinine clearance levels from this population and calculated 95% confidence intervals on each of those samples, the true creatinine clearance level for the population would fall inside about 950 of the intervals we calculated.

ATTACK RATES

When you read the newspaper, you might notice that journalists refer to epidemics or outbreaks and use the term **attack rate**. Attack rates are used to determine the origin of an outbreak, particularly with foodborne illnesses. You calculate the attack rate by taking all those exposed to the agent of interest and putting that number in the denominator. You then consider, of this group, who got sick and put that number in the numerator. Finally, to make it a percentage you multiply by 100. (That should sound familiar: It is the incidence rate for the exposed group, which is your relative risk numerator. See how these terms relate?)

$$\text{Attack rate} = \frac{\text{Cases in the exposed group} \left(\text{those who got sick}\right)}{\text{All those exposed to that particular agent}} \times 100$$

Let's look at an example. The health department is investigating an outbreak of salmonella and has determined that many of those with positive stool cultures were at a wedding with 200 people in attendance 2 days earlier. When health department employees interview those at the wedding about what they ate, they determine the information shown in **Table 13-2**.

You can see the attack rates that are associated with the individual food items in the table. The health department investigation team will use this type of table to determine the probable source of the contamination—from this data, it is likely to be the alfalfa sprouts because they have the highest attack rate. The health department will now follow up this piece of information with some additional testing to make a final determination about the cause of the outbreak.

These calculations probably seem very simple, but they can trick you if you are not careful. I always start with the denominator, which

may seem a little backward, but that is where most students make their mistake. The denominator of an attack rate is *all* those exposed to the agent, which includes those who are sick and those who are well. When attempting to calculate an attack rate for the caviar, many students want to start with the number of people who ate the caviar and got sick (which is the correct numerator), but then they put the number of people who ate the caviar and were well in the denominator, or they put the whole population in the denominator. (Notice that not everyone at the wedding ate the caviar, so 200 is not the denominator.) I find that starting with the denominator is the best way to avoid this issue. If you begin with who was exposed, it helps remind you to include everyone who ate that particular food. You can then go back and figure out, *of that group*, how many subjects got sick.

Let's try another example. Out of 203 party guests, 27 ate goulash, 36 ate lasagna, and 87

TABLE 13-2	**Attack Rates, Table 1**			
Exposure of Interest	**Number Sick Who Consumed This Item**	**Number Well Who Consumed This Item**	**Total Number Who Consumed This Item**	**Attack Rate**
Caviar	2	45	47	$\frac{2}{47} \times 100 = 4.3\%$
Alfalfa sprouts	18	24	42	$\frac{18}{42} \times 100 = 42.9\%$
Hummus	1	12	13	$\frac{1}{13} \times 100 = 7.7\%$
Roast beef	5	43	48	$\frac{5}{48} \times 100 = 10.4\%$
Chicken	6	32	38	$\frac{6}{38} \times 100 = 15.8\%$

TABLE 13-3	**Attack Rates, Table 2**			
Exposure of Interest	**Number Sick Who Consumed This Item**	**Number Well Who Consumed This Item**	**Total Number Exposed to This Item**	**Attack Rate**
Goulash	10	17	27	
Lasagna	7	29	36	
Shrimp	30	57	87	
Alcohol	unknown	unknown	180	

ate shrimp. One hundred and eighty guests consumed alcohol. Seventeen people were sick the next day, including 10 who ate goulash, 7 who ate lasagna, and 30 who ate shrimp.

To use attack rates to determine the likely source of the outbreak, the first thing you need to do is determine the denominator of each attack rate, which I am sure you remember is the number of people who were exposed (or consumed) each item (see **Table 13-3**).

Let's fill in the last column together.

- The attack rate for the goulash was 10/27, which means that, of the 27 people who ate goulash, 10 were sick. This equals 37%.
- The attack rate for lasagna was 7/36, which means that, of the 36 people who ate lasagna, 7 got sick. This equals 19%.
- The attack rate for shrimp was 30/87, which means that, of the 87 people who ate shrimp, 30 got sick. This equals 34%.

We cannot determine the attack rate for the alcohol consumption because, although we know the denominator (the number at risk) is 180, we don't know how many of them got sick.

We cannot simply add the number who are sick because some of them may be counted in multiple categories. For example, a person who had a shrimp appetizer followed by lasagna and then got sick the next day is counted in both the number who got sick and ate shrimp and the number who got sick and ate lasagna. You can also see that not everyone at the party (203) drank alcohol, so we don't know if someone who didn't drink alcohol and got sick is included in the total number of those who are sick.

Notice that the highest attack rate is associated with the goulash. The item with the highest attack rate is the likely source of the outbreak, so in this situation, something in the goulash was the likely source. Notice that although more people who ate shrimp got sick, it is a lower attack rate because a lot of people ate shrimp and didn't get sick. You cannot look only at the absolute numbers; you have to look at percentages.

Sometimes you know the attack rate and need to estimate how many cases are likely to develop in order to allocate resources effectively or plan for necessary prevention and control. For example, if a virus has an attack rate of 10% and there are 45,000 susceptible people in the region under consideration, you would anticipate approximately 4,500 cases. Having an idea of how many people are likely to become sick is very helpful knowledge for public health planning and response.

Case Control Study

A cohort study sounds great, but what about when you can't get a grant to cover the cost of a 40-year prospective trial? Or you are trying to finish a dissertation in less than 40 years? Or if you want to examine a disease that is incredibly rare and may not even show up in a sample of 300 even if you follow them for 40 years? Another study design frequently used in epidemiology, especially when funding is tight or the disease is rare, is called a **case control study**. This type of study starts with the outcome of interest (the disease) and looks back to determine exposure. For example, 10 patients in your hospital have a rapidly progressing case of respiratory failure. All 10 were relatively healthy adults until developing symptoms that included fever and a cough.

You may start your study with this as your sample population (10 cases with similar unusual symptoms) and look back to determine what they may have been exposed to. You interview the patients and their families; review their medical records; and collect data on food consumed, recent travel, occupational exposures, previous illnesses, sexual partners, drug use, and living situations. You also obtain biological specimens. Unfortunately, because you start with those who are already ill (prevalence cases), you cannot calculate an incidence (new cases) rate. However, you can still calculate an approximation of the relative risk, which is the **odds ratio (OR)**: an estimate of the risk of *being* sick, not *becoming* sick (Kahn & Sempos, 1989).

Let's continue with your study of the 10 patients with the unknown disease causing respiratory failure. In addition to your sample of 10 sick patients, you select 10 healthy controls from the community. After completing your interviews and chart reviews, you see that six of the sick patients recently traveled to Eastern Asia and

TABLE 13-4	**Exposure to Birds and Respiratory Failure**		
	Cases	**Controls**	**Total**
Exposure	$A = 8$	$B = 4$	12
No exposure	$C = 2$	$D = 6$	8
Total	10	10	20

lived in villages where wild birds were raised among the community. Two others worked in a chicken processing plant. Four of your healthy controls also had some type of bird exposure but were not sick. You decide to calculate an OR to see what association may be found between the illness and exposure to some type of bird. You set up another 2 × 2 table (see **Table 13-4**).

Because this is a case control study, you calculate an OR that divides the odds that a case was exposed by the odds that a control was exposed. Odds and probability are two different things. Odds are the chances that something happens divided by the chance that it doesn't. For example, if the probability of your passing an exam is 80%, the chance that you won't is 20%. The odds of your passing the exam are 80% ÷ 20%, or 4:1 (Gordis, 2000).

To calculate the odds of a case being exposed using a 2 × 2 table, divide *A* by *C*. In the example, this would be 8 ÷ 2; in plain English, the odds that a sick patient was exposed to birds are 4:1. The odds of a control being exposed are *B* ÷ *D*, or 4 ÷ 6, or 0.66. To get the odds ratio, take 4 ÷ 0.66 to get 6.06. The odds are six times higher that a case (sick patient) was exposed to the birds than a healthy control was. You can do a bit of math and determine that the equation can actually be simplified to

$$\frac{AD}{BC}$$

In this example:

$$\frac{8 \times 6}{4 \times 2} = 6$$

If you find that version easier, you are welcome to do it. If you hate to memorize things (as I do), think about what the OR means, and figure out the math from there.

You will see OR and RR used more frequently in the public health and nursing literature because they are easier for the general public to understand. If you are using the OR to estimate the RR, you can then report that your study *estimates* that individuals exposed to the birds are six times as likely to be sick or that exposure to the birds is associated with an estimated six fold increase in the risk of developing this illness. If these results are significant, they can help the investigator determine the possible causative agent for the respiratory failure by prompting funding for a cohort study or for further investigation. They can also be used to convey public health concerns to the public in a readily understandable way.

You may recall logistic regression, which is the form of regression utilized when the outcome is binary, or has only two possibilities, such as alive or dead. One of the reasons researchers like to use logistic regression is that, with a little math, the beta values in the prediction equation can be converted to odds ratios. When you see the SPSS output for a logistic regression model, you will see a column titled Exp(B). This column indicates the odds ratio associated with that particular exposure and the outcome of interest. Let's consider an example. If a study involving 10,000 subjects reports that having diabetes, having high cholesterol, smoking, and age all affect the probability of being dead upon arrival at a hospital emergency room, you might see a table such as the one in **Table 13-5.**

The last column in the table is Exp(B), which is the exponentiation of the beta coefficient, otherwise known as the odds ratio for that particular independent variable when all the others are held constant. In other words, having diabetes means a subject is 1.576 times as likely to be dead upon arrival compared to subjects who do not have diabetes when all the other independent variables are held constant, or remain the same. In this same example, each yearly increase in age increases the chance of

TABLE 13-5	**Factors Relating to the Chance of Being Dead upon Arrival in a Hospital Emergency Room ($N = 10,000$)**					
Variables in the Equation	B	S.E.	Wald	df	Sig.	Exp(B)
Diabetes	0.455	0.097	21.888	1	0.000	1.576
cholesterol	0.453	0.059	59.295	1	0.000	1.574
Smoking	0.471	0.065	52.743	1	0.000	1.602
Age	0.030	0.003	88.204	1	0.000	1.031
Constant	−4.124	0.212	377.786	1	0.000	0.016

B = beta coefficient; S.E. = standard error; Wald = a type of chi-square test; df = degrees of freedom; Sig. = significance of the Wald chi-square; Exp(B) = odds ratio.

being dead upon arrival 1.03 times. Again, being able to report an OR is helpful when you are trying to explain complicated research to the general public, so someday you, too, may find yourself using logistic regression.

Also, when using the OR to estimate the RR, the results are most accurate when the cases are rare (10% incidence or prevalence), and the cases and controls should be representative of the population in terms of the exposure of interest (Sullivan, 2008). Don't forget that the OR is an estimate of the RR, not the same thing; so if you are using this tool incorrectly, your results may not be meaningful.

CROSS-SECTIONAL STUDY

The last type of study frequently used in epidemiology literature is a **cross-sectional study**, which collects the data about exposure and outcome at the same time. For example, suppose you surveyed the nurses on your unit and asked them how many hours they worked that day and if they were tired. You would have data but not a time sequence. All the data is collected at the same time. This is a significant limiting factor because you cannot determine the direction of the relationship even if you find one. For example, in a survey about work hours and fatigue, you might hypothesize that the hours a nurse works is associated with fatigue; however, with a cross-sectional survey, you cannot assume that the hours worked came before the fatigue. What if the nurse actually came to work fatigued because her spouse is out of work and she deals with a lot of stress at home? She may still work an extra shift that is requested because she needs the additional income, but her fatigue actually started before she came to

work. You don't know whether the fatigue is related to the hours worked or to preexisting factors or to factors that contributed to the decision to work extra hours. Cross-sectional studies offer preliminary results and can be useful in forming hypotheses, but they are usually only the beginning of the examination of any significant research issue.

ATTRIBUTABLE RISK

Attributable risk is another concept that makes sense to most nonstatisticians and therefore is a helpful tool when you are disseminating public health information. **Attributable risk for the exposed group (AR_e)** tells you the amount of a disease or outcome in an exposed group that is due to a particular exposure. It is very easy to calculate. The formula is:

$$AR_e = \text{Incidence rate in the exposed group}$$
$$- \text{Incidence rate in the nonexposed group}$$

For example, let's say you develop a cohort study to examine the relationship between tanning bed usage and cataract development. You put your results in the 2×2 table shown in **Table 13-6**. The incidence rate for the exposed group is 60 per 100. The incidence rate for the unexposed group is 10 per 100. (This is what is considered background risk, or the risk for everyone who does not have the exposure you are looking at.) The attributable risk for the exposed group is the difference: 60/100 − 10/100 = 50/100, or 50 cases per 100 individuals. If tanning beds were eliminated, you could prevent up to 50 cases of cataracts for 100 individuals who would have tanned before this new policy. (Of course, they could just hit

TABLE 13-6	Tanning Bed Exposure and Cataract Development		
	Cataracts	No Cataracts	Total
Tanning bed usage	60	40	100 (exposed)
No tanning	10	90	100 (nonexposed)
Totals	70 (diseased)	130 (nondiseased)	200

the beaches and lay out in the sun; this is why you can only say *up to* 50 cases.)

To make this number meaningful, determine the proportion of the excess risk (beyond background risk) that is associated with exposure to tanning beds by dividing 50 by 60 (the incidence in the exposed group): The result is 0.83, or 83%. This tells you how much of the risk of cataracts is due to tanning beds in those who used the tanning beds.

How could you use this information clinically? You might advise your patients who tan that, if they stop using the tanning beds, they could reduce their risk of developing cataracts by 83%. Most patients will understand this information much more easily than if you start talking about incidence and relative risk (Gordis, 2000). It is also the type of information that large populations can understand and that is meaningful to public officials, not to mention making a great headline!

SUMMARY

You have now completed this chapter and should be feeling very confident with this material. To review some key concepts, let's start with epidemiology. Epidemiology is the study of the distribution of disease. Three types of epidemiological studies are the cohort study, case control study, and cross-sectional study.

A cohort study is done by following a group of individuals over time to see who develops the outcome of interest. Remember to exclude prevalence cases in this design because they already have the trait you are studying or wish to study. The incidence data you collect allows you to determine the number of new cases among your sample during the duration of your study.

The relative risk is the incidence rate in the exposed sample divided by the incidence rate of those not exposed. The incidence rate in the exposed sample is the definition of an attack rate. Attack rates are useful in outbreak investigations and can be calculated for many different agents or exposures of interest.

A protective effect occurs anytime you have a significant relative risk less than one. A relative risk of one means that there is no association between the exposure and the illness. An exposure is considered an associated risk factor for the disease when the relative risk is greater than one. Remember, for any exposure to be a significant risk or protective factor, the *p*-value must be less than alpha, or the confidence limits must be entirely above or entirely below 1.

A case control study involves starting with the outcome of interest and working backward to determine exposure. The odds ratio is used to calculate the approximation of the relative risk. You must have incidence data to calculate a relative risk. The odds ratio uses prevalence data (those who are already sick) and estimates relative risk.

In a cross-sectional design, you collect data about exposure and outcomes at the same time.

Public health information has to be delivered in a way that the general public can understand. The results discussed in this chapter may help convert research results into meaningful information for the media and for the general public. People need to be able to understand the important clinical information you have worked so hard to determine!

These new concepts will be helpful to you in mastering statistics, particularly if you are interested in becoming an epidemiologist (a blatant plug for epidemiology).

CHAPTER 13 REVIEW QUESTIONS

Questions 1–9: The variables in **Table 13-7** have been examined to determine the association with length of labor.

TABLE 13-7   **Variables Related to Length of Labor >12 Hours**

Variable	RR	95% CI	*p*-Value
Maternal age <40			
Yes	0.87	(0.721.23)	0.23
No (reference group)	1.00		
Support person present			
Yes	0.43	(0.310.56)	0.03
No (reference group)	1.00		
Previous birth			
Yes	0.21	(0.180.24)	0.01
No (reference group)	1.00		
Epidural anesthesia			
Yes	1.20	(1.061.34)	0.02
No anesthesia or IV/IM anesthesia (reference group)	1.00		

1.   What are your "exposure" or independent variables?

2. What is your outcome or dependent variable?

3. Instead you measure your dependent variable rounded to the nearest full hour. What level of measurement is it? Is it quantitative or qualitative?

4. Suppose you originally measured this variable as a yes-or-no response to the question, "Did you feel as though you had a very long labor?" What level of measurement was it? Was it a quantitative or qualitative question?

5. If the study has an alpha of 0.05, which variables are associated with the length of labor? Which are associated with a decreased length of labor? Which are associated with an increased length of labor?

6. Note that when the *p*-value is significant, the RR confidence intervals do not include the value of one. Why?

7. Did maternal age significantly increase the risk of having a labor greater than 12 hours?

8. Did using epidural anesthesia significantly increase the risk of having a longer labor? Compared to whom?

9. Interpret in plain English the RR for maternal age and length of labor.

10. A study reports that children who have breakfast are more likely to pass the fourth-grade math competency (RR = 1.39, 95% CL = 1.30–1.49). Because the 95% confidence limits do not include an RR of 1, your know that these results are:

TABLE 13-8	**Factors Related to Risk of Falling Asleep 2 Hours after Exposure**	
Variable	**RR**	**95% CI**
Caffeine	0.67	0.550.75
Melatonin	1.34	1.211.46
Exercise	0.88	0.701.18
Television	0.93	0.890.99

Questions 11–15: A sleep disorder clinic conducted a small cohort study with medical residents working 24-hour shifts to examine how exposure to caffeine, melatonin, strenuous exercise, or television affects the risk of medical residents falling asleep 2 hours later. The results are shown in **Table 13-8**.

11. What factors are significantly related to the risk of the residents falling asleep?

12. What is the dependent or outcome variable?

13. Which exposure had the greatest positive impact on the risk of falling asleep 2 hours after exposure?

14. Interpret the RR for television. Is it significant?

15. Which exposure was most effective in decreasing the risk of falling asleep 2 hours later?

Questions 16–17: The small cohort study with medical residents was replicated, but this time the researchers examined the effect of these exposures on sleep 6 hours later. See **Table 13-9**.

16. Offer a reasonable explanation for the data in the table.

TABLE 13-9	**Factors Related to Risk of Falling Asleep 6 Hours after Exposure**	
Variable	**RR**	**95% CI**
Caffeine	0.89	0.541.51
Melatonin	1.02	0.801.45
Exercise	1.34	1.172.08
Television	0.96	0.890.99

TABLE 13-10	**Alcohol Use and Traumatic Injury in Adolescent Males**		
	Traumatic Injury	**No Traumatic Injury**	**Totals**
Alcohol use	98	40	138
No alcohol use	10	52	61
Totals	108	92	200

17. A taxi company wants to implement a policy to diminish the risk of falling asleep behind the wheel. The company has the greatest number of accidents due to drivers falling asleep on the evening shift between 9 p.m. and 11 p.m. The company is considering either opening the company gym for use by the cab drivers between 1 p.m. and 3 p.m. or making free coffee available during the dinner hour (6 p.m.–7 p.m.). Which policy would the research about the risk of falling asleep support implementing?

Questions 18–20: A cohort study following a group of 200 randomly selected adolescent males finds the results shown in **Table 13-10**.

18. Calculate the incidence rate for traumatic injury.

19. What is the attributable risk for the exposed group? Interpret the risk in plain English.

20. Calculate the RR of traumatic injury for adolescent males who consume alcohol. Assuming your RR is significant, interpret this value.

Questions 21–26: A preschool class visited the zoo. As part of the trip, they had a chance to pet a large lizard and then had lunch. Some students brought lunch from home; others bought lunch at the zoo. That evening four students became ill.

21. What is the attack rate associated with petting the lizard?

22. What is the attack rate associated with bringing lunch from home?

23. What is the attack rate associated with buying lunch at the zoo?

24. Is petting the lizard, lunch from home, or lunch from the zoo the likely source of the contamination? Explain your answer.

25. If petting the lizard is the source of the contamination, how do you explain student number 7?

TABLE 13-11	**Exposure and Disease Status for Preschool Investigation**		
Student	**Pet the Lizard**	**Lunch**	**Sick**
1	Yes	Home	Yes
2	No	Home	No
3	No	Home	No
4	Yes	Zoo	Yes
5	Yes	Home	Yes
6	No	Zoo	No
7	Yes	Home	No
8	Yes	Zoo	Yes

26. If there were a student who got sick but did not pet the lizard, does this mean petting the lizard is not the source of contamination? What other explanations could there be?

_____

_____

Questions 27–33: You are an infectious disease expert interested in determining if administering tuberculosis (TB) treatment with a directly observed therapy (DOT) program has an impact on the risk of developing multiple-drug-resistant (MDR) tuberculosis. You randomly select 120 individuals newly diagnosed with TB and randomize them into two equal groups—one group receives treatment without DOT, and one group receives treatment with DOT. You follow the groups for 2 years and identify all cases of MDR TB that develop. You find that 2 of the individuals who receive treatment and DOT develop MDR TB, and 10 of the individuals who receive treatment without DOT develop MDR TB.

27. Is this a probability or nonprobability sample?

_____

_____

28. Instead of randomly assigning the groups into those who receive DOT and those who do not, the researcher identified a group that received DOT and a group that did not and observed the two groups for a period of 10 years to see who developed MDR TB. What type of epidemiologic or observational study design is this study?

_____

_____

_____

29. Complete the appropriate 2 × 2 table.

_____

_____

30. What is the RR of developing MDR TB?

_____

_____

31. Interpret the RR in plain English.

_____

_____

32. Say that the 95% CL was 0.12–0.45. Is this result significant?

_____

_____

33. Is DOT a risk factor or a protective factor?

_____

_____

Questions 34–37: There is an outbreak of a highly infectious virus in your region that is associated with an attack rate of 22% among adults ages 18–65, 43% in those over age 65, and 31% among children < 18 years.

	Regional Population	Attack Rate	Anticipated Number of Cases
Children < 18 years	68,430		
Adults 18–65	190,000		
Elderly > 65	87,000		

34. Use the following information to determine the anticipated number of cases you will see in each age category in your region.
35. What is the total number of cases you should anticipate in your region?
36. Which age group will likely have the largest number of cases? Why?
37. Most of the children who are infected with this virus require hospitalization and ventilator support for 5–7 days. Your region currently has 167 pediatric-compatible ventilators. Does this concern you at all? Why?

Research Application Article

Read the following article to see how several researchers assessed the RR of nosocomial infections before and after a handwashing intervention. These concepts will make more and more sense to you as you see them used in actual clinical research.

Chhapola, V., & Brar, R. (2015). Impact of an educational intervention on hand hygiene compliance and infection rate in a developing country neonatal intensive care unit. *International Journal of Nursing Practice, 21*(5), 486–492. doi:10.1111/ijn.12283

1. What type of sample was utilized for this study?
2. The study states it has a quasi-experimental design. Why is this not a randomized control trial?
3. During the study, no other new infection control procedures were implemented. How would this affect the validity of the study?
4. If a new antibiotic policy were started before this study, how might a carryover effect have impacted the results?
5. In this study, data for each observed opportunity for handwashing was recorded as correctly performed or not (yes or no). What level of measurement is this variable?
6. Instead the data were collected as the number of errors made while handwashing. The variable would be at what level of measurement?
7. Look at table 1 in the article. What was the rate of health care workers' (HCWs') performance of correct handwashing techniques between patient encounters before and after the intervention?
8. Look at table 1 in the article. A chi-square test is completed to determine if there is an increase in correct handwashing technique between patient encounters. Was there a significantly significant relationship between the variables? Explain.
9. Look at table 1 in the article. Interpret the RR that HCWs correctly wash their hands between patient encounters.
10. Look at table 1 in the article. Were HCWs significantly more likely to wash their hands correctly after leaving the patient?

11. Look at table 1 in the article. After the intervention, were the HCWs significantly more likely to wash their hands correctly after removing gloves?

12. Look at table 2 in the article. Which types of HCW had a significant increase in correct handwashing after the intervention?

13. Look at table 2 in the article, where the incidence rates for nosocomial infections per 100 neonatal admissions were calculated. What percentage developed a nosocomial infection in this unit before and after the handwashing intervention?

14. Look at table 2 in the article, where the incidence rates for nosocomial infections per 100 neonatal admissions were calculated. If an infant were admitted to the Neonatal Intensive Care Unit (NICU) after the intervention, what would be the RR of developing a nosocomial infection when compared to admission before the intervention?

15. The authors of the article indicate there may have been a Hawthorne Effect in this study because the participants knew they were being observed after phase 1. If that is true, what might happen to correct handwashing once the observers are no longer at the site?

16. If these studies were replicated in other developing nations and the intervention was simple and inexpensive to implement, would you recommend this intervention? Why or why not?

17. What might you suggest to measure any Hawthorne Effect occurring in the study?

ANSWERS TO ODD-NUMBERED CHAPTER 13 REVIEW QUESTIONS

1. Maternal age < 40, having a support person present, previous births, and epidural anesthesia

3. Interval, quantitative

5. Having a support person present (decreased risk of labor >12 hours), having had previous births (decreased risk of labor > 12 hours), and using epidural anesthesia (increased risk of labor > 12 hours)

7. No, RR is not significant.

9. Answers will vary. For example, maternal age less than 40 years is not significantly associated with the risk of labor > 12 hours.

11. Caffeine, melatonin, television

13. Melatonin increased falling asleep 2 hours later.

15. Caffeine

17. Free coffee! Exercise 6 hours before going on shift would increase the number of times the cab drivers fell asleep, whereas coffee 2 hours before the shift would decrease it.

19. Fifty-five out of 100 of the cases of injuries in adolescent men are in adolescents who consume alcohol.

21. 4/5, or 80%

23. 2/3, or 66.7%

25. Answers will vary. They may include that the student may have washed his or her hands, or his or her immune system may have been strong enough to destroy any contamination ingested.

27. Probability sample

29.

	Disease Positive	No Disease	Row Totals
Exposure to DOT	2	58	60
No exposure	10	50	60
Column totals	12	108	120

31. The group who received DOT was less likely (or only 20% as likely) to develop MDR TB compared to those who did not receive DOT. If you would rather put it in terms of not having DOT, those who did not have DOT were 5.57 [RR = (10/60)/(2/60)] times as likely to develop MDR TB compared to those who did receive DOT.

33. A protective exposure

35. 100,423

37. Answers will vary. They may include: Yes, although we don't know how quickly the children will become sick, if there are

21,213 sick children who need ventilators for 5–7 days and only 167 pediatric-compatible ventilators, the turnover of ventilators as pediatric patients recover or pass away may not be adequate, and we may run out of pediatric ventilators.

Research Application Article

1. A convenience sample included all HCWs at the site.

3. Keeping other factors that could also affect the outcome from changing during the study would improve the validity or accuracy of the study.

5. Nominal

7. 47% to 74%

9. RR = 1.56 (1.51–1.62). Because the 95% CI is always over the value of 1, we know that the intervention was significantly associated with higher levels of the outcome variable. This means that the HCWs are significantly more likely to wash their hands correctly after the intervention.

11. No. The RR is 1.25; however, the 95% CI is 0.87–1.78, which includes the value of one. Thus, the corresponding p-value is not significant because within the 95% CI is the possibility that the intervention increased, did not affect, or decreased the amount of correct handwashing episodes.

13. 46% to 21%

15. There might be a decrease in correct handwashing again.

17. Conduct another follow-up observation made at a point when the participants do not know they are being monitored.

APPENDIX A

TABLES FOR REFERENCE

| TABLE 1 | *t* Table. Table Entries Are Values of *t* Random Variables.* |

Cumulative probability	0.75	0.80	0.85	0.90	0.95	0.975	0.99	0.995	0.9975	0.999	0.9995
Upper-tail probability	0.25	0.20	0.15	0.10	0.05	0.025	0.01	0.005	0.0025	0.001	0.0005

Degrees of freedom											
1	1.000	1.376	1.963	3.078	6.314	12.71	31.82	63.66	127.3	381.3	636.6
2	0.816	1.061	1.386	1.886	2.920	4.303	6.965	9.925	14.09	22.33	31.60
3	0.765	0.978	1.250	1.638	2.353	3.182	4.541	5.841	7.453	10.21	12.92
4	0.741	0.941	1.190	1.533	2.132	2.776	3.747	4.604	5.598	7.173	8.610
5	0.727	0.920	1.156	1.476	2.015	2.571	3.365	4.032	4.773	5.893	6.869
6	0.718	0.906	1.134	1.440	1.943	2.447	3.143	3.707	4.317	5.208	5.959
7	0.711	0.896	1.119	1.415	1.895	2.365	2.998	3.499	4.029	4.785	5.408
8	0.706	0.889	1.108	1.397	1.860	2.306	2.896	3.355	3.833	4.501	5.041
9	0.703	0.883	1.100	1.383	1.833	2.262	2.821	3.250	3.690	4.297	4.781
10	0.700	0.879	1.093	1.372	1.812	2.228	2.764	3.169	3.581	4.144	4.587
11	0.697	0.876	1.088	1.363	1.796	2.201	2.718	3.106	3.497	4.025	4.437
12	0.695	0.873	1.083	1.356	1.782	2.179	2.681	3.055	3.428	3.930	4.318
13	0.694	0.870	1.079	1.350	1.771	2.160	2.650	3.012	3.372	3.852	4.221
14	0.692	0.868	1.076	1.345	1.761	2.145	2.624	2.977	3.326	3.787	4.140
15	0.691	0.866	1.074	1.341	1.753	2.131	2.602	2.947	3.286	3.733	4.073
16	0.690	0.865	1.071	1.337	1.746	2.120	2.583	2.921	3.252	3.686	4.015
17	0.689	0.863	1.069	1.333	1.740	2.110	2.567	2.898	3.222	3.646	3.965
18	0.688	0.862	1.067	1.330	1.734	2.101	2.552	2.878	3.197	3.610	3.922

(continues)

| TABLE 1 | *t* Table. Table Entries Are Values of *t* Random Variables.* (*Continued*) | | | | | | | | | | |

Cumulative probability	0.75	0.80	0.85	0.90	0.95	0.975	0.99	0.995	0.9975	0.999	0.9995
Upper-tail probability	0.25	0.20	0.15	0.10	0.05	0.025	0.01	0.005	0.0025	0.001	0.0005
19	0.688	0.861	1.066	1.328	1.729	2.093	2.539	2.861	3.174	3.579	3.883
20	0.687	0.860	1.064	1.325	1.725	2.086	2.528	2.845	3.153	3.552	3.850
21	0.686	0.859	1.063	1.323	1.721	2.080	2.518	2.831	3.135	3.527	3.819
22	0.686	0.858	1.061	1.321	1.717	2.074	2.508	2.819	3.119	3.505	3.792
23	0.685	0.858	1.060	1.319	1.714	2.069	2.500	2.807	3.104	3.485	3.768
24	0.685	0.857	1.059	1.318	1.711	2.064	2.492	2.797	3.091	3.467	3.745
25	0.684	0.856	1.058	1.316	1.708	2.060	2.485	2.787	3.078	3.450	3.725
26	0.684	0.856	1.058	1.315	1.706	2.056	2.479	2.779	3.067	3.435	3.707
27	0.684	0.855	1.057	1.314	1.703	2.052	2.473	2.771	3.057	3.421	3.690
28	0.683	0.855	1.056	1.313	1.701	2.048	2.467	2.763	3.047	3.408	3.674
29	0.683	0.854	1.055	1.311	1.699	2.045	2.462	2.756	3.038	3.396	3.659
30	0.683	0.854	1.055	1.310	1.697	2.042	2.457	2.750	3.030	3.385	3.646
40	0.681	0.851	1.050	1.303	1.684	2.021	2.423	2.704	2.971	3.307	3.551
60	0.679	0.848	1.045	1.296	1.671	2.000	2.390	2.660	2.915	3.232	3.460
80	0.678	0.846	1.043	1.292	1.664	1.990	2.374	2.639	2.887	3.195	3.416
100	0.677	0.845	1.042	1.290	1.660	1.984	2.364	2.626	2.871	3.174	3.390
1000	0.675	0.842	1.037	1.282	1.646	1.962	2.330	2.581	2.813	3.098	3.300
z	0.674	0.842	1.036	1.282	1.645	1.960	2.326	2.576	2.807	3.090	3.291
Confidence level	50%	60%	70%	80%	90%	95%	98%	99%	99.5%	99.8%	99.9%

The left margin of the table is labeled **Degrees of freedom**.

*t values computed with Microsoft Excel 9.0 TINV function.

TABLE 2

F Table. Table Entries Are *F* Values with Right-Tail Probability *P*.*

	P	\multicolumn{11}{c}{Degrees of freedom in numerator (df_1)}
	P	1	2	3	4	5	6	7	8	12	24	1000
---	---	---	---	---	---	---	---	---	---	---	---	---
1	0.100	39.86	49.50	53.59	55.83	57.24	58.20	58.91	59.44	60.71	62.00	63.30
	0.050	161.4	199.5	215.7	224.6	230.2	234.0	236.8	238.9	243.9	249.1	254.2
	0.025	647.8	799.5	864.2	899.6	921.8	937.1	948.2	956.7	976.7	997.2	1017.7
	0.010	4052	4999	5403	5625	5764	5859	5928	5981	6106	6235	6363
	0.001	405284	499999	540379	562500	576405	585937	592873	598144	610668	623497	6363011
2	0.100	8.53	9.00	9.16	9.24	9.29	9.33	9.35	9.37	9.41	9.45	9.49
	0.050	18.51	19.00	19.16	19.25	19.30	19.33	19.35	19.37	19.41	19.45	19.49
	0.025	38.51	39.00	39.17	39.25	39.30	39.33	39.36	39.37	39.41	39.46	39.50
	0.010	98.50	99.00	99.17	99.25	99.30	99.33	99.36	99.37	99.42	99.46	99.50
	0.001	998.50	999.00	999.17	999.25	999.30	999.33	999.36	999.37	999.42	999.46	999.50
3	0.100	5.54	5.46	5.39	5.34	5.31	5.28	5.27	5.25	5.22	5.18	5.13
	0.050	10.13	9.55	9.28	9.12	9.01	8.94	8.89	8.85	8.74	8.64	8.53
	0.025	17.44	16.04	15.44	15.10	14.88	14.73	14.62	14.54	14.34	14.12	13.91
	0.010	34.12	30.82	29.46	28.71	28.24	27.91	27.67	27.49	27.05	26.60	26.14
	0.001	167.03	148.50	141.11	137.10	134.58	132.85	131.58	130.62	128.32	125.93	123.53
4	0.100	4.54	4.32	4.19	4.11	4.05	4.01	3.98	3.95	3.90	3.83	3.76
	0.050	7.71	6.94	6.59	6.39	6.26	6.16	6.09	6.04	5.91	5.77	5.63
	0.025	12.22	10.65	9.98	9.60	9.36	9.20	9.07	8.98	8.75	8.51	8.26
	0.010	21.20	18.00	16.69	15.98	15.52	15.21	14.98	14.80	14.37	13.93	13.47
	0.001	74.14	61.25	56.18	53.44	51.71	50.53	49.66	49.00	47.41	45.77	44.09
5	0.100	4.06	3.78	3.62	3.52	3.45	3.40	3.37	3.34	3.27	3.19	3.11
	0.050	6.61	5.79	5.41	5.19	5.05	4.95	4.88	4.82	4.68	4.53	4.37

Degrees of freedom in denominator (df_2)

(continues)

TABLE 2

F Table. Table Entries Are F Values with Right-Tail Probability P. (Continued)

df₂	P	\multicolumn{11}{c}{Degrees of freedom in numerator (df_1)}

df_2	P	1	2	3	4	5	6	7	8	12	24	1000
	0.025	10.01	8.43	7.76	7.39	7.15	6.98	6.85	6.76	6.52	6.28	6.02
	0.010	16.26	13.27	12.06	11.39	10.97	10.67	10.46	10.29	9.89	9.47	9.03
	0.001	47.18	37.12	33.20	31.09	29.75	28.83	28.16	27.65	26.42	25.13	23.82
6	0.100	3.78	3.46	3.29	3.18	3.11	3.05	3.01	2.98	2.90	2.82	2.72
	0.050	5.99	5.14	4.76	4.53	4.39	4.28	4.21	4.15	4.00	3.84	3.67
	0.025	8.81	7.26	6.60	6.23	5.99	5.82	5.70	5.60	5.37	5.12	4.86
	0.010	13.75	10.92	9.78	9.15	8.75	8.47	8.26	8.10	7.72	7.31	6.89
	0.001	35.51	27.00	23.70	21.92	20.80	20.03	19.46	19.03	17.99	16.90	15.77
7	0.100	3.59	3.26	3.07	2.96	2.88	2.83	2.78	2.75	2.67	2.58	2.47
	0.050	5.59	4.74	4.35	4.12	3.97	3.87	3.79	3.73	3.57	3.41	3.23
	0.025	8.07	6.54	5.89	5.52	5.29	5.12	4.99	4.90	4.67	4.41	4.15
	0.010	12.25	9.55	8.45	7.85	7.46	7.19	6.99	6.84	6.47	6.07	5.66
	0.001	29.25	21.69	18.77	17.20	16.21	15.52	15.02	14.63	13.71	12.73	11.72
8	0.100	3.46	3.11	2.92	2.81	2.73	2.67	2.62	2.59	2.50	2.40	2.30
	0.050	5.32	4.46	4.07	3.84	3.69	3.58	3.50	3.44	3.28	3.12	2.93
	0.025	7.57	6.06	5.42	5.05	4.82	4.65	4.53	4.43	4.20	3.95	3.68
	0.010	11.26	8.65	7.59	7.01	6.63	6.37	6.18	6.03	5.67	5.28	4.87
	0.001	25.41	18.49	15.83	14.39	13.48	12.86	12.40	12.05	11.19	10.30	9.36
9	0.100	3.36	3.01	2.81	2.69	2.61	2.55	2.51	2.47	2.38	2.28	2.16
	0.050	5.12	4.26	3.86	3.63	3.48	3.37	3.29	3.23	3.07	2.90	2.71
	0.025	7.21	5.71	5.08	4.72	4.48	4.32	4.20	4.10	3.87	3.61	3.34
	0.010	10.56	8.02	6.99	6.42	6.06	5.80	5.61	5.47	5.11	4.73	4.32
	0.001	22.86	16.39	13.90	12.56	11.71	11.13	10.70	10.37	9.57	8.72	7.84

Degrees of freedom in denominator (df_2)

Degrees of freedom in numerator (df_1)

df_2													
10	0.100	3.29	2.92	2.73	2.61	2.52	2.46	2.41	2.38	2.28	2.18	2.06
	0.050	4.96	4.10	3.71	3.48	3.33	3.22	3.14	3.07	2.91	2.74	2.54
	0.025	6.94	5.46	4.83	4.47	4.24	4.07	3.95	3.85	3.62	3.37	3.09
	0.010	10.04	7.56	6.55	5.99	5.64	5.39	5.20	5.06	4.71	4.33	3.92
	0.001	21.04	14.91	12.55	11.28	10.48	9.93	9.52	9.20	8.45	7.64	6.78
12	0.100	3.18	2.81	2.61	2.48	2.39	2.33	2.28	2.24	2.15	2.04	1.91
	0.050	4.75	3.89	3.49	3.26	3.11	3.00	2.91	2.85	2.69	2.51	2.30
	0.025	6.55	5.10	4.47	4.12	3.89	3.73	3.61	3.51	3.28	3.02	2.73
	0.010	9.33	6.93	5.95	5.41	5.06	4.82	4.64	4.50	4.16	3.78	3.37
	0.001	18.64	12.97	10.80	9.63	8.89	8.38	8.00	7.71	7.00	6.25	5.44
14	0.100	3.10	2.73	2.52	2.39	2.31	2.24	2.19	2.15	2.05	1.94	1.80
	0.050	4.60	3.74	3.34	3.11	2.96	2.85	2.76	2.70	2.53	2.35	2.14
	0.025	6.30	4.86	4.24	3.89	3.66	3.50	3.38	3.29	3.05	2.79	2.50
	0.010	8.86	6.51	5.56	5.04	4.69	4.46	4.28	4.14	3.80	3.43	3.02
	0.001	17.14	11.78	9.73	8.62	7.92	7.44	7.08	6.80	6.13	5.41	4.62
16	0.100	3.05	2.67	2.46	2.33	2.24	2.18	2.13	2.09	1.99	1.87	1.72
	0.050	4.49	3.63	3.24	3.01	2.85	2.74	2.66	2.59	2.42	2.24	2.02
	0.025	6.12	4.69	4.08	3.73	3.50	3.34	3.22	3.12	2.89	2.63	2.32
	0.010	8.53	6.23	5.29	4.77	4.44	4.20	4.03	3.89	3.55	3.18	2.76
	0.001	16.12	10.97	9.01	7.94	7.27	6.80	6.46	6.19	5.55	4.85	4.08
18	0.100	3.01	2.62	2.42	2.29	2.20	2.13	2.08	2.04	1.93	1.81	1.66
	0.050	4.41	3.55	3.16	2.93	2.77	2.66	2.58	2.51	2.34	2.15	1.92
	0.025	5.98	4.56	3.95	3.61	3.38	3.22	3.10	3.01	2.77	2.50	2.20
	0.010	8.29	6.01	5.09	4.58	4.25	4.01	3.84	3.71	3.37	3.00	2.58
	0.001	15.38	10.39	8.49	7.46	6.81	6.35	6.02	5.76	5.13	4.45	3.69

(continues)

Degrees of freedom in denominator (df_2)

TABLE 2

F Table. Table Entries Are F Values with Right-Tail Probability P. (Continued)

df₂	P	\multicolumn{11}{c}{Degrees of freedom in numerator (df₁)}

Degrees of freedom in denominator (df₂)	P	1	2	3	4	5	6	7	8	12	24	1000
20	0.100	2.97	2.59	2.38	2.25	2.16	2.09	2.04	2.00	1.89	1.77	1.61
	0.050	4.35	3.49	3.10	2.87	2.71	2.60	2.51	2.45	2.28	2.08	1.85
	0.025	5.87	4.46	3.86	3.51	3.29	3.13	3.01	2.91	2.68	2.41	2.09
	0.010	8.10	5.85	4.94	4.43	4.10	3.87	3.70	3.56	3.23	2.86	2.43
	0.001	14.82	9.95	8.10	7.10	6.46	6.02	5.69	5.44	4.82	4.15	3.40
30	0.100	2.88	2.49	2.28	2.14	2.05	1.98	1.93	1.88	1.77	1.64	1.46
	0.050	4.17	3.32	2.92	2.69	2.53	2.42	2.33	2.27	2.09	1.89	1.63
	0.025	5.57	4.18	3.59	3.25	3.03	2.87	2.75	2.65	2.41	2.14	1.80
	0.010	7.56	5.39	4.51	4.02	3.70	3.47	3.30	3.17	2.84	2.47	2.02
	0.001	13.29	8.77	7.05	6.12	5.53	5.12	4.82	4.58	4.00	3.36	2.61
50	0.100	2.81	2.41	2.20	2.06	1.97	1.90	1.84	1.80	1.68	1.54	1.33
	0.050	4.03	3.18	2.79	2.56	2.40	2.29	2.20	2.13	1.95	1.74	1.45
	0.025	5.34	3.97	3.39	3.05	2.83	2.67	2.55	2.46	2.22	1.93	1.56
	0.010	7.17	5.06	4.20	3.72	3.41	3.19	3.02	2.89	2.56	2.18	1.70
	0.001	12.22	7.96	6.34	5.46	4.90	4.51	4.22	4.00	3.44	2.82	2.05
100	0.100	2.76	2.36	2.14	2.00	1.91	1.83	1.78	1.73	1.61	1.46	1.22
	0.050	3.94	3.09	2.70	2.46	2.31	2.19	2.10	2.03	1.85	1.63	1.30
	0.025	5.18	3.83	3.25	2.92	2.70	2.54	2.42	2.32	2.08	1.78	1.36
	0.010	6.90	4.82	3.98	3.51	3.21	2.99	2.82	2.69	2.37	1.98	1.45
	0.001	11.50	7.41	5.86	5.02	4.48	4.11	3.83	3.61	3.07	2.46	1.64

Degrees of freedom in numerator (df_1)

1000											
0.100	2.71	2.31	2.09	1.95	1.85	1.78	1.72	1.68	1.55	1.39	1.08
0.050	3.85	3.00	2.61	2.38	2.22	2.11	2.02	1.95	1.76	1.53	1.11
0.025	5.04	3.70	3.13	2.80	2.58	2.42	2.30	2.20	1.96	1.65	1.13
0.010	6.66	4.63	3.80	3.34	3.04	2.82	2.66	2.53	2.20	1.81	1.16
0.001	10.89	6.96	5.46	4.65	4.14	3.78	3.51	3.30	2.77	2.16	1.22

*F values computed with Microsoft Excel 9.0 FINV function.

TABLE 3	**Chi-Square Table.***

	Probability in Right Tail									
df	0.975	0.25	0.20	0.15	0.10	0.05	0.025	0.01	0.005	0.001	0.0005
1	0.00098	1.32	1.64	2.07	2.71	3.84	5.02	6.63	7.88	10.83	12.12
2	0.051	2.77	3.22	3.79	4.61	5.99	7.38	9.21	10.60	13.82	15.20
3	0.216	4.11	4.64	5.32	6.25	7.81	9.35	11.34	12.84	16.27	17.73
4	0.48	5.39	5.99	6.74	7.78	9.49	11.14	13.28	14.86	18.47	20.00
5	0.83	6.63	7.29	8.12	9.24	11.07	12.83	15.09	16.75	20.52	22.11
6	1.24	7.84	8.56	9.45	10.64	12.59	14.45	16.81	18.55	22.46	24.10
7	1.69	9.04	9.80	10.75	12.02	14.07	16.01	18.48	20.28	24.32	26.02
8	2.18	10.22	11.03	12.03	13.36	15.51	17.53	20.09	21.95	26.12	27.87
9	2.70	11.39	12.24	13.29	14.68	16.92	19.02	21.67	23.59	27.88	29.67
10	3.25	12.55	13.44	14.53	15.99	18.31	20.48	23.21	25.19	29.59	31.42
11	3.82	13.70	14.63	15.77	17.28	19.68	21.92	24.72	26.76	31.26	33.14
12	4.40	14.85	15.81	16.99	18.55	21.03	23.34	26.22	28.30	32.91	34.82
13	5.01	15.98	16.98	18.20	19.81	22.36	24.74	27.69	29.82	34.53	36.48
14	5.63	17.12	18.15	19.41	21.06	23.68	26.12	29.14	31.32	36.12	38.11
15	6.26	18.25	19.31	20.60	22.31	25.00	27.49	30.58	32.80	37.70	39.72
16	6.91	19.37	20.47	21.79	23.54	26.30	28.85	32.00	34.27	39.25	41.31
17	7.56	20.49	21.61	22.98	24.77	27.59	30.19	33.41	35.72	40.79	42.88
18	8.23	21.60	22.76	24.16	25.99	28.87	31.53	34.81	37.16	42.31	44.43
19	8.91	22.72	23.90	25.33	27.20	30.14	32.85	36.19	38.58	43.82	45.97
20	9.59	23.83	25.04	26.50	28.41	31.41	34.17	37.57	40.00	45.31	47.50
21	10.28	24.93	26.17	27.66	29.62	32.67	35.48	38.93	41.40	46.80	49.01
22	10.98	26.04	27.30	28.82	30.81	33.92	36.78	40.29	42.80	48.27	50.51
23	11.69	27.14	28.43	29.98	32.01	35.17	38.08	41.64	44.18	49.73	52.00
24	12.40	28.24	29.55	31.13	33.20	36.42	39.36	42.98	45.56	51.18	53.48
25	13.12	29.34	30.68	32.28	34.38	37.65	40.65	44.31	46.93	52.62	54.95
26	13.84	30.43	31.79	33.43	35.56	38.89	41.92	45.64	48.29	54.05	56.41
27	14.57	31.53	32.91	34.57	36.74	40.11	43.19	46.96	49.64	55.48	57.86
28	15.31	32.62	34.03	35.71	37.92	41.34	44.46	48.28	50.99	56.89	59.30
29	16.05	33.71	35.14	36.85	39.09	42.56	45.72	49.59	52.34	58.30	60.7

df	Probability in Right Tail										
	0.975	0.25	0.20	0.15	0.10	0.05	0.025	0.01	0.005	0.001	0.0005
30	16.79	34.80	36.25	37.99	40.26	43.8	47.0	50.9	53.7	59.7	62.2
40	24.43	45.62	47.27	49.24	51.81	55.76	59.34	63.69	66.77	73.40	76.09
50	32.36	56.33	58.16	60.35	63.17	67.50	71.42	76.15	79.49	86.66	89.56
60	40.48	66.98	68.97	71.34	74.40	79.08	83.30	88.38	91.95	99.61	102.69
80	57.15	88.13	90.41	93.11	96.58	101.88	106.63	112.33	116.32	124.84	128.26
100	74.22	109.1	111.7	114.7	118.5	124.3	129.6	135.8	140.2	149.4	153.2

*Chi-square values computed with Microsoft Excel 9.0 CHINV function.

WORKING WITH SMALL SAMPLES

Dr. Renee Biedlingmaier

WORKING WITH SMALL SAMPLE SIZES

Having a large enough sample helps to ensure the internal and external validity of research studies. However, gaining access to subjects is often challenging. For example, if a researcher investigates the impact of an intervention in long-term-care facilities, access to staff at these facilities is necessary. After accessing the staff, investigators have to identify those who are willing to spend time taking part in the study. Long-term-care facilities do not generally have staff with extra time in their workday beyond their work duties, so this may further limit the sample size. Unfortunately, collecting a sizable sample may not be feasible. However, determining the utility of the intervention may still be of value in order to avoid spending time and financial resources on an intervention that is not effective. Thus, it is important that researchers working with small samples appropriately select statistical analyses and mindfully determine the potential impact of the small sample size on the study results.

VIOLATION OF ASSUMPTIONS DUE TO SMALL SAMPLES

To make inferences about a population from a sample, that sample must be comprised of characteristics representative of the population of interest. Large randomized samples offer the best opportunity to limit sampling error and selection bias (Polit & Beck, 2012). There are many statistical tests to choose from, each of which incorporates assumptions about population attributes. Depending on the statistical test, these attributes vary. Random sampling is usually desirable; it helps ensure that the characteristics represented in the population of interest have an equivalent opportunity of being present in the study sample (Polit & Beck, 2012). Researchers can use parametric tests, such as independent or dependent sample *t*-tests, analysis of variance (ANOVA), or repeat-measures analysis of variance, with normally or nearly normally distributed dependent variables measured at the interval or ratio level (Polit & Beck, 2012).

What should be done, however, if you have a small and potentially nonrandomized sample? In this situation, there are different types of statistical analyses to consider using. There is a decreased likelihood of a normal distribution of dependent variables with a small and possibly nonrandomized sample, making nonparametric analyses a better option. Nonparametric tests exclude the assumption that the data are normally distributed (Polit & Beck, 2012). Although parametric analyses have greater power, nonparametric tests are often the appropriate option when working with small and/or nonrandomized samples. We will investigate power in more detail a little later.

STATISTICAL TESTS USED IN NURSING WHEN SAMPLES ARE SMALL

When there is a violation of assumptions such as randomization and/or normality of distribution for parametric tests, nonparametric tests are used. The basis for appropriate test selection is the level of measurement for the dependent variable and the number and type of comparison groups. When violation of the normality assumption is a concern, the table in next column can help guide test selection.

SMALL SAMPLES: LIMITATIONS IN STUDY INTERPRETATION

Some challenges with interpretation of results arise when studies havev small samples. Let's review a few of the potential problems. Sample size and confidence interval size are inversely

Statistical Test	Number/Type of Groups Being Compared	Dependent Variable— Level of Measurement
Spearman's rank-order correlation	Single-group	Ordinal/interval/ratio
Chi-square test	2/independent	Nominal
Man-Whitney U	2/independent	Ordinal
t-test	2/Independent	Interval/ratio
Chi-square	More than 2/independent	Nominal
Kruskal-Wallis test	More than 2/independent	Ordinal
ANOVA	More than 2/independent	Interval/ratio
Paired t-test	2/dependent	Nominal
Wilcoxon signed-ranks test	2/dependent	Ordinal
McNemar's test	2/dependent	Interval/ratio
RM-ANOVA	More than 2/Dependent	Nominal
Friedman	More than 2/Dependent	Ordinal
Cochran's Q	More than 2/Dependent	Interval/ratio

Data from Polit, D.F. & Beck, C.T. (2012). *Nursing research: Generating and assessing evidence for nursing practice.* (9th ed.). Philadelphia: Wolters Kluwer Health/Lippincott Williams & Wilkins.

proportional. Smaller sample sizes mean wider confidence intervals. Wider confidence intervals lead to a less precise estimate of the population mean. Hence, researchers must account for the impact of sample size when conducting analyses with estimated distributions (Polit & Beck, 2012).

Conducting a sample size calculation prior to starting a research study (a priori) can help ensure there is a sufficient sample and reduce the risk that results are simply due to chance. Small samples increase the risk of making a type two error. If there is a small difference between group means or ranks of scores, a small sample may not have enough power to reveal that difference. When this happens, investigators may erroneously fail to reject the null hypothesis and miss a difference when one exists (type two error).

REAL-WORLD APPLICATION

In the beginning of this section, we indicated that research questions might still be important and worth attempting to study even when only small samples are feasible. In these situations, investigators assess and discuss the impact of small samples on the validity of study results when interpreting the findings.

SMALL SAMPLE WITH INCONCLUSIVE RESULTS

During an investigation of the impact of an educational intervention on the knowledge, skills, and attitudes about oral care of demented institutionalized elderly, obtaining the minimal sample of 78 participants with an alpha of .05 and a power of 80 for a paired or dependent samples *t*-test proved to be challenging at best. The study included two long-term-care facilities, each with between 90 and 100 certified nurse assistants. Despite multiple mitigating actions, the resultant sample fell far short of the minimum of 78, with an ultimate sample size of 13.

Due to the final sample size of 13, the investigators were not able to analyze between-facility data using independent samples *t*-tests, thus

diminishing the reliability of findings. Due to the lack of normal distribution of data, utilization of the nonparametric Wilcoxon signed ranks for paired data replaced the paired or dependent samples *t*-test for within-facility analyses. No significant differences were identified (see the table below).

Wilcoxon Signed Ranks Comparisons of Questions—Long-Term-Care Study

	Wilcoxon Signed Ranks
n = 13	*p*
5 questions SH	−.315 (.478)
5 questions RB	−.197 (.720)

Note: SH = systemic health, RB = resistant behaviors, *p*-value = .05

Ultimately, a post hoc power analysis revealed a power of .29, indicating that this was a significantly underpowered study with great risk of a type two error. Thus, the researchers assessed that unless the educational intervention made a large difference, the sample was too small to identify the difference, and they were not able to determine if the intervention was or was not effective in changing knowledge, skills, and attitudes about oral care of demented institutionalized elderly.

SMALL SAMPLE WITH SIGNIFICANT RESULTS

In contrast, Rosner, Glynn, and Lee (2007) did a study investigating the relationship between intraocular pressure (IOP) and grade of retinopathy. Contrary to the previously referenced study, the researchers found statistically significant results using a similar nonparametric Wilcoxon signed rank sum test for non-normally distributed data. In the table below is a brief overview of their statistically significant results:

Wilcoxon Signed Rank Sum Test Examples

IOP Comparison Results	Wilcoxon Signed Rank Sum Test
	p
Right eye ($n = 71$)	2.344 (.019)*
Left eye ($n = 61$)	−1.822 (.069)
All eyes	2.339 (.019)*

* Statistically significant results ($p <$ alpha). Data from Rosner, B., Glynn, R. J., & Lee, M-L.T. (2007). A nonparametric test for observational non-normally distributed ophthalmic data with eye-specific exposures and outcomes. *Ophthalmic Epidemiology, 14*, pp. 243–250. doi:10.1080/09286580701396704

SUMMARY

Small samples create challenges. Sometimes researchers can utilize statistical techniques to accommodate the small sample. In other situations, however, the small samples produce too great of a risk of a type two error to draw a reasonably certain conclusion. It is important for researchers to understand the limitations created by small samples and the appropriate statistical tests to utilize before analyzing and interpreting data and results.

REFERENCES

Agresti, A. (2002). *Categorical data analysis* (2nd ed.). Wiley Series in Probability and Statistics. Hoboken, NJ: Wiley.

Anifantaki, S., Prinianakis, G., Vitsaksaki, E., Katsouli, V., Mari, S., Symianakis, A., et al. (2009). Daily interruption of sedative infusions in an adult medical-surgical intensive care unit: Randomized controlled trial. *Journal of Advanced Nursing, 65*(5), 1054–1060.

Barthel, C., Wiegand, S., Scharl, S., Scharl, M., Frei, P., Vavricka, S. R., & . . . Biedermann, L. (2015). Patients' perceptions on the impact of coffee consumption in inflammatory bowel disease: Friend or foe?—A patient survey. *Nutrition Journal, 14*(1), 1–8. doi:10.1186/s12937-015-0070-8

Chhapola, V., & Brar, R. (2015). Impact of an educational intervention on hand hygiene compliance and infection rate in a developing country neonatal intensive care unit. *International Journal of Nursing Practice, 21*(5), 486-492. doi:10.1111/ijn.12283

Chen, M., Shiao, Y., & Gau, Y. (2007). Comparison of adolescent health-related behavior in different family structures. *Journal of Nursing Research, 15*(1), 1–10.

Chhapola, V., & Brar, R. (2015). Impact of an educational intervention on hand hygiene compliance and infection rate in a developing country neonatal intensive care unit. *International Journal of Nursing Practice, 21*(5), 486–492. doi:10.1111/ijn.12283

Chung, Y. C., & Hwang, H. L. (2008). Education for homecare patients with leukemia following a cycle of chemotherapy: An exploratory pilot study [online exclusive]. *Oncology Nursing Forum, 35*(5), E86–E87.

Corless, I., Lindgren, T., Holzemer, W., Robinson, L., Moezzi, S., Kirksey, K., et al. (2009). Marijuana effectiveness as an HIV self-care strategy. *Clinical Nursing Research, 18*(2), 172–193.

Corty, E. W. (2007). *Using and interpreting statistics: A practical text for the health, behavioral and social sciences.* St. Louis, MO: Mosby.

Doering, L., Cross, R., Magsarili, M., Howitt, L., & Cowan, M. (2007). Utility of observer-rated and self-report instruments for detecting major depression in women after cardiac surgery. *American Journal of Critical Care, 16*(3), 260–269.

Gordis, L. (2000). *Epidemiology* (2nd ed.). Philadelphia, PA: W. B. Saunders.

Grove, S. K. (2007). *Statistics for health care research: A practical workbook.* St. Louis, MO: W. B. Saunders.

Heyman, H., Van De Looversosch, D., Jeijer, E., & Schols, J. (2008). Benefits of an oral nutritional supplement on pressure ulcer healing in long-term care. *Journal of Wound Care, 17*(11), 476–480.

Johnson, N. L., & Kotz, S. (1997). *Leading personalities in statistical sciences.* Wiley Series in Probability and Statistics. Hoboken, NJ: Wiley.

Kahn, H., & Sempos, C. (1989). *Statistical methods in epidemiology.* New York, NY: Oxford University Press.

Khan, H. A., Sobki, S. H., & Alhomida, A. S. (2015). Regression analysis for testing association between fasting blood sugar and glycated hemoglobin in diabetic patients. *Biomedical Research, 26*(3), 604–606.

Mosfeldt, M., Pedersen, O. B., Riis, T., Worm, H. O., van Mark, S., Jørgensen, H. L., . . . Lauritzen, J. B. (2012). Value of routine blood tests for prediction of mortality risk in hip fracture patients. *Acta Orthopaedica, 83*(1), 31–35. http://doi.org/10.3109/17453674.2011.652883

Munro, B. H. (2005). *Statistical methods for health care research* (5th ed.). Philadelphia, PA: Lippincott Williams & Wilkins.

New York State Nurses Association. (n.d.). *Mandatory overtime law.* Retrieved from http://www.nysna .org/practice/mot/intro.htm

Nieswiadomy, R. (2008). *Foundations of nursing research* (5th ed.). Upper Saddle River, NJ: Pearson Education.

Norman, G. R., & Streiner, D. L. (2008). *Biostatistics: The bare essentials* (3rd ed.). Hamilton, ON, Canada: BC Decker.

Oepkes, D., Seaward, P. G., Vandenbussche, F. P., Windrim, R., Kingdom, J., Bevene, J., et al. (2006). Doppler ultrasonography versus amniocentesis to predict fetal anemia. *New England Journal of Medicine, 355*(2), 156–164.

Olbrys, K. M. (2001). The effect of topical lidocaine anesthetic on reported pain in women who undergo needle wire localization prior to breast biopsy. *Southern Online Journal of Nursing Research, 6*(2), 1–18.

Özden, D., & Görgülü, R. S. (2015). Effects of open and closed suction systems on the haemodynamic parameters in cardiac surgery patients. *Nursing in Critical Care, 20*(3), 118–125. doi:10.1111/nicc.12094

Pagano, M., & Gauvreau, K. (1993). *Principles of biostatistics.* Belmont, CA: Wadsworth.

Papastavrou, E., Tsangari, H., Kalokerinou, A., Papacostas, S., & Sourtzi, P. (2009). Gender issues in caring for demented relatives. *Health Science Journal, 3*(1), 41–53.

Plichta, S. B., & Garzon, L. S. (2009). *Statistics for nursing and allied health.* Philadelphia, PA: Wolters Kluwer Health/Lippincott Williams & Wilkins.

Polit, D. F., & Beck, C. T. (2012). *Nursing research: Generating and assessing evidence for nursing practice* (9th ed.). Philadelphia, PA: Wolters Kluwer Health/Lippincott Williams & Wilkins.

Rosner, B., Glynn, R. J., & Lee, M-L.T. (2007). A nonparametric test for observational non-normally distributed ophthalmic data with eye-specific exposures and outcomes. *Ophthalmic Epidemiology, 14,* 243–250. doi:10.1080/09286580701396704

Scherer, Y. K., Foltz-Ramos, K., Fabry, D., & Chao, Y-Y. (2016). Evaluating simulation methodologies to determine best strategies to maximize student learning. *Journal of Professional Nursing, 32*(5), 349-357. doi:10.1016/j.profnurs.2016.01.003

Schilling, F., Spix, C., Berthold, F., Erttmann, R., Fehse, N., Hero, B., et al. (2002). Neuroblastoma screening at one year of age. *New England Journal of Medicine, 346*(14), 1047–1053.

Sullivan, L. M. (2008). *Essentials of biostatistics in public health.* Sudbury, MA: Jones & Bartlett.

Tobian, A., Serwadda, D., Quinn, T. C., Kigozi, G., Gravitt, P. E., Laeyendecker, O., et al. (2009). Male circumcision for the prevention of HSV2 and HPV infection and syphilis. *New England Journal of Medicine, 360*(13), 1298–1309.

Tukey, J. W. (1977). *Exploratory data analysis.* Retrieved from http://pdfs.semanticscholar.org

Tussey, C. M., Botsios, E., Gerkin, R. D., Kelly, L. A., Gamez, J., & Mensik, J. (2015). Reducing length of labor and cesarean surgery rate using a peanut ball for women laboring with an epidural. *The Journal of Perinatal Education, 24*(1), 16–24. doi:10.1891/1058-1243.24.1.16

Vassiliadou, A., Stamatopoulou, E., Triantafyllou, G., Gerodimou, E., Toulia, G., & Pistolas, D. (2008). The role of nurses in the sexual counseling of patients after myocardial infarction. *Health Science Journal, 2*(2), 111–118.

Watson, J., Kinstler, A., Vidonish III, W. P., Wagner, M., Li, L., Davis, K. G., . . . Daraiseh, N. M. (2015). Impact of noise on nurses in pediatric intensive care units. *American Journal of Critical Care, 24*(5), 377–384. doi:10.4037/ajcc2015260

Zellner, K., Boerst, C., & Tabb, W. (2007). Statistics used in current nursing research. *Journal of Nursing Education, 46*(2), 55–59.

Zurmehly, J. (2008). The relationship of educational preparation, autonomy, and critical thinking to nursing job satisfaction. *Journal of Continuing Education in Nursing, 39*(10), 453–460.

EPILOGUE

You've completed the book—I know there is a collective sigh of relief happening right now! I hope you are more comfortable and confident in your ability to understand statistics. You've successfully covered a lot of material and have mastered a great deal of math and statistical concepts. Even if you started this course with some trepidation, I hope you now see that you are quite capable of mastering the statistics you have learned throughout this course. I hope you also realize that statistics can be helpful to your practice as a nurse and that you have the potential to contribute to the growing need for evidence-based practice in our profession. I hope this text helped make the process as painless as possible, and that someday you, too, may become a nurse who "crunches numbers" to help care for your patients in the best way possible. Thank you for allowing me to join you on this journey. I wish you all the best as you go forth in your professional nursing career.

Beth

INDEX

A

adjusted *R*-squared, 208, 228
alpha, 100, 102, 114, 116, 149, 152
alternative hypothesis, 100, 101, 128, 149, 152, 172, 180
analysis of variance (ANOVA), 172
   alternative hypothesis, 172
   carry-over effects, 172, 176, 181
   comparing more than two samples, 172
   compound symmetry, 172, 177
   degrees of freedom, Student *t*-test, 174
   distribution, relationship between, 175
   F-statistic calculation, 178
   homogeneity of variance, 149, 155, 159, 172, 175, 177
   issues of concern with, 176–177
   null hypothesis, 172–173
   position or latency effects, 172, 176
   repeat-measures, 172, 176–177, 181
   statistical significance, 174–175
   table, 179–180, 224, 229, 237
   use of, 175–176
ANOVA. *See* analysis of variance
attack rate, 250, 260–262
attributable risk, 265–266
   for exposed group, 250, 265

B

bar chart, 20, 23–28, 158
beta, 114, 117, 121
bimodal, 42, 43, 57
bivariate normal, 195
box and whiskers plot, 20, 30–31
   central tendency and range, to display, 47–48

C

carry-over effects, 172, 176, 181
case control study, 250, 263–265
categorical data analysis, 130
categorical dependent variable, 231
categorical variables, 2, 6, 178

central limit theorem, 88–90
central tendency, 42, 57
   box and whiskers plot, 47–48
   defined, 43
   measures of, 43–44
chi-square, 129–132
   distribution, 175
   when not to use, 132
   test, 128, 135, 192, 193, 198, 255
clinical significance, 100, 104–106
cluster sampling, 84, 86, 93
coefficient of determination, 192, 195, 199
coefficients table, 230
cohort study, 250–257, 266
comparing more than two samples, 172
compound symmetry, 172, 177
confidence intervals, 257–258
content validity, 64, 65
contingency table, 68
continuous variable, 2, 6, 178
convenience sampling, 84, 91, 93
convergent validity, 64, 65
correlation, 192, 198
correlation coefficient, 64, 195–198
   alternative hypothesis, 192–193
   bivariate normal, 195
   chi-square test, 192, 193
   coefficient of determination, 192, 195, 199
   correlation, 192, 198
   correlation test selection, 193
   direction of relationship, 192, 193–194
   homoscedasticity, 192, 195
   null hypothesis, 192–193
   Pearson's correlation coefficient, 192, 193, 195
   percentage of variance, 192, 195–196, 199
   sample size, 194
   Spearman's correlation coefficient, 192
   statistical significance, 194
   strength of relationship, 192, 194
   use of, 195

criteria
  exclusion, 84, 92–93
  inclusion, 84, 92–93
Cronbach's alpha, 64, 67
crossover clinical trial, 155
cross-sectional study, 250, 265
cumulative frequency, 20, 21, 23, 49
cumulative percentage, 20, 23, 31
cumulative relative frequency, 20, 21

D
data presentation
  bar chart, 20, 23–28, 158
  cumulative frequency, 20, 21, 49
  cumulative percentage, 20, 23, 31
  frequency distribution, 20–22, 23, 51–54
  frequency table, 25
  grouped frequency, 20, 22
  histogram, 20, 28–29, 31
  line graph, 20, 29
  outlier, 20, 30, 44, 57
  percentage, 20, 22–23
    calculating, 22
    defined, 22
  percentile rank, 20, 23
  percentiles, 20, 24
    calculation formula, 26
  quantiles, 24
  quartiles, 20, 24
  scatterplot, 20, 29–30
degrees of freedom, Student *t*-test, 128, 129, 146, 152–154, 174
  formula for calculating, 153
denominator of sample variance, 46–47
dependent samples, 146, 147, 176, 181
dependent variable, 2, 5–6, 160, 176, 181, 209
descriptive statistics, 42, 157
determination coefficient, 192, 195, 199
direction of relationship, 129–130, 192
discrete variables, 6
distribution, relationship between, 175
divergent validity, 64, 65, 74

E
effect size, 114–115, 121
efficiency (EFF), 64, 74–75
  calculation formula, 74
empirical method, 2, 3, 11
epidemiology, 250–265

equivalence, 64, 67
error, 119, 121
  type one, 114, 118–119
  type two, 114, 117–118
estimate, 2, 4
exclusion criteria, 84, 92–93
extreme outlier, 42

F
F-statistic calculation, 178
fail to reject the null hypothesis, 100, 101
feasibility, 64, 65
frequency distribution, 20–22, 23, 31, 42, 51
  vs. probability distributions, 51–54
frequency table, 25, 45, 49, 60, 156

G
grouped frequency, 20, 22, 31

H
histogram, 20, 28–29, 31
homogeneity, 64, 66, 74
  of variance, 149, 155, 159, 172, 175
hypothesis, 100
  alternative, 100, 101, 172
  null, 100, 101, 107–108, 172–173
hypothesis testing, 100–102
  steps, 105

I
incidence cases, 250, 251, 254
inclusion criteria, 84, 92–93
independent samples, 128, 132, 146, 172, 176
independent variable, 2, 5–6, 209, 218, 228–229
  to regression model, 233
inferential statistics, 51, 54
inter-rater reliability, 64, 67
internal consistency reliability, 64, 67
interval data, 2, 9

L
latency effects, 172, 176, 181
level of measurement, 6–9, 146–151
Levene's test for equality of variances, 146, 159, 160
line graph, 20, 29, 31
linear regression, 208, 209
logistic regression, 208, 231, 264–265

M

McNemar test, 132
mean, 42, 44, 160
measurement levels, 6–9, 146–151
measurement tool evaluation, 63–82
    efficiency, 74
    negative predictive value, 73–74
    positive predictive value, 71–73
    reliability, 64, 66–68
    screening tests, 68–69
    sensitivity, 69
    specificity, 69–70
measures of central tendency, 43–44, 57
median, 42, 44, 54, 57
mode, 42, 43, 54, 57
multimodal, 42, 44, 57
multinomial logistic regression, 231
multiple regression, 208, 214, 231–238

N

negative predictive value (NPV), 64, 73–74
nominal data, 2, 7, 28, 43, 44
noninferiority trial, 146, 149
nonprobability sampling, 84, 90–92
    in qualitative research, 92
    types of, 91–92
        convenience sampling, 91
        quota sampling, 91–92
normal curve, 106
normal distribution, 42, 54–56
    changing mean, 55
    changing variance, 56
    defined, 54, 55
    probability and, 49
normal equations, 219
normal error linear regression model, 217
normal error regression model, 211, 217
normal error simple linear regression model, 219
NPV. *See* negative predictive value
null hypothesis, 100, 101, 107–108, 128, 149,
        172–173, 192

O

odds ratio (OR), 208, 231, 250, 263, 264, 266
one-tailed test, 149
OR. *See* odds ratio
ordinal data, 2, 9, 44, 193
ordinary least squares, 219
outlier, 20, 30, 44, 56–57

P

parameter, 2, 4, 55
    estimates, 219–223
Pearson's chi-square test, 130–132
    by hand, 133
Pearson's correlation coefficient, 192, 193,
        195, 198
percentage, 20, 22–23
    calculating, 22
    defined, 22
percentage of variance, 192, 195–196, 199
percentile rank, 20, 23
percentiles, 20, 24
    calculation formula, 26
population, 2, 4
    defined, 4
    vs. sample, 4
position or latency effects, 172, 176, 181
positive predictive value (PPV), 64, 71–73
    calculation formula, 71
power, 114–115, 118, 119, 152, 172, 176
power analysis, 114, 119, 121
power errors, 117
PPV. *See* positive predictive value
prediction error, 214
predictive validity, 64, 65
predictive value
    negative, 64, 73–74
    positive, 71–73
prevalence, 64, 71
prevalence cases, 250, 251
probability, 2, 4, 42, 49
    and normal distribution, 49
probability distribution, 42, 51–54, 175
probability sampling, 84–86
    cluster sampling, 86
    simple random sampling, 85
    stratified sampling, 86
    systematic sampling, 85–86
protective effect, 250, 254, 266

Q

qualitative measure, 2, 4
qualitative research, nonprobability
        sampling in, 92
quantiles, 24
quantitative measure, 2, 4
quartiles, 20, 24
quota sampling, 84, 91–92

R

R-squared change, 208, 229
R-squared (*R*²) value, 208, 224–228, 238
range, 42, 44–45
   box and whiskers plot, 47–48
ratio data, 2, 9, 57, 193
regression, 208
regression analysis, quantifying an association, 208–239
regression coefficient, 208, 214, 218
   calculation, 219–223
regression line, 225, 226
regression model, 211, 233
   equation, 218, 223
reject the null hypothesis, 100, 101
relationship
   direction of, 192, 193–194
   strength of, 194, 198–199
relative frequency, 20, 21, 49
relative risk (RR), 250, 251, 253, 266
   interpretations of, 254
relative risk of one, 250, 255
reliability, 64, 66–68, 74
repeat-measures ANOVA, 172, 176–177, 181
   defined, 176
   issues of concern with, 176–177
   use of, 177
research idea
   alpha, 100, 102
   alternative hypothesis, 100, 101
   clinical significance, 100, 104–106
   hypothesis, 100
   hypothesis testing, 100–102
      steps, 105
   normal curve, 106
   null hypothesis, 100, 101, 107–108
   statistical significance, 100, 102–103
   statistical testing, 105
   type one error, 100, 102
residual, 208, 214, 215
   calculation, 217
   and error, 217
risk factor, 250, 255, 256
risk ratio, 250, 251
RR. *See* relative risk

S

sample, 2, 4
sample size, 92–93, 114, 116, 119–121, 194
sample variance, 46–47
sampling bias, 84, 86

sampling distribution, 42, 54, 84, 87
sampling error, 84, 146, 152
   defined, 86
   vs. sampling bias, 86–87
sampling methods, 84–85
   central limit theorem, 88–90
   exclusion criteria, 92–93
   inclusion criteria, 92–93
   nonprobability sampling, 90–92
      in qualitative research, 92
      types of, 91–92
   probability sampling, 85–86
      cluster sampling, 86
      simple random sampling, 85
      stratified sampling, 86
      systematic sampling, 85–86
   sampling bias, 86
   sampling distribution, 84, 87
   sampling error, 84, 86
      vs. sampling bias, 86–87
   standardized scores, 88
scale variable, 55
scatterplot, 20, 29–30
screening test, 68–69, 71
sensitivity, 64, 68–69, 71
   calculation formula, 69
   and specificity, 69–70
simple random sampling, 84, 85, 93
skewed distribution, 42, 56–57
Spearman correlation coefficient, 192, 193, 198
specificity, 64, 69–70, 75
   calculation formula, 69
   sensitivity and, 69–70
SSE. *See* sum of squares due to error
SSR. *See* sum of squares due to regression
SSTO. *See* total sum of squares
stability, 64, 66, 74
standard deviation, 42, 45
   calculating, 45–46
   range and, 44–45
standard error of estimate, 208, 228
standardized scores, 88
standard normal variable, calculation
      formula, 56
statistical model, 211
statistical relationship, 211
statistical significance, 100, 102–103, 108, 129,
      152, 174–175, 194
   vs. clinical significance, 104–106
   defined, 102
statistical testing, 105

statistics, 2
  definition of, 3, 4
stratified sampling, 84, 86, 93
strength of relationship, 192, 194, 199
Student *t*-test, 146, 147
  alternative hypothesis, 152
  degrees of freedom, 146, 152–154
    formula for calculating, 153
  dependent samples, 146
  independent samples, 146
  level of measurement, 146–151
  methods, 155
  noninferiority trial, 146, 149
  null hypothesis, 152
  one-tailed test, 149
  statistical significance, 152
  two-tailed test, 152
study designs used in epidemiology, 251–265
sum of squares, 219
  concept of, 220
  due to error (SSE), 225, 226
    calculation, 227
    formula, 236
  due to regression (SSR), 225, 226
    ANOVA table for, 237
    calculation, 227
    formula, 236
systematic sampling, 84, 85–86, 93

T

t-statistical distribution, 155
t-test, Student. *See* Student *t*-test

test statistic, 107
total sum of squares (SSTO), 225, 226
  ANOVA table for, 236
  calculation, 226, 235
transformation, 175
trendline, 212–214
Tukey fences, 42, 48, 57
2 × 2 table, 68, 71, 128
two-tailed test, 152
type one error, 100, 102, 114, 118–119
type two error, 114, 117–118, 121

U

unimodal, 43

V

validity, 65–66, 74
  content, 64, 65
  convergent, 64, 65
  divergent, 64, 65, 74
  predictive, 64, 65
variable, 2, 4
  properties of, 42
variance analysis. *See* analysis of variance
variance, homogeneity of, 149, 155, 159, 175, 177

Z

Z-score, 57, 107